MENTAL HEALTH, RECLAIMED

PRAISE FOR MENTAL HEALTH, RECLAIMED

In this vulnerable and important book, Dr. Azi lays out the disturbing state of affairs for modern medicine's system of diagnosis and treatment. She then gives us a vision for how we can reclaim our health and wellness through practical and sensible methodologies. This book is as eye-opening as it is uplifting.

—Dr. Edith Eger,
NYT Bestselling Author, World Renowned
Trauma Psychologist, & Holocaust Survivor

Drawing from her own journey through bipolar disorder and extensive research, Dr. Azi Jankovic presents a holistic framework addressing the physiological, psychological, social, and spiritual dimensions of healing—precisely the approach needed to transform our understanding of mental health. Her innovative ECHO method (Education, Curiosity, Healing, Observation) empowers readers to reclaim agency through nutrition, sleep, movement, and meaningful connection, proving that a diagnosis can become a doorway to deeper healing and genuine thriving rather than a life sentence.

—Ellen Vora, MD.
Board Certified, Holistic Psychiatrist
and Author of The Anatomy of Anxiety

"Dr. Azi's journey is not only inspiring but also a touchstone for anyone striving to find balance and healing in the face of mental health challenges."

—Ben Epstein Ph.D,
Clinical Psychologist and Author of Living in the Presence

Azi's radical honesty throughout these pages is an inspiration for anyone seeking to better their lives, understand themselves, and challenge negative and confining narratives around mental health. This book opens up a new way of healing for whole-person mental health and wellbeing.

—Nomi Spain-Levy,
CNS, MS Nutrition & Functional Medicine, Double Board-Certified Nutritionist & Health Coach

Mental Health, Reclaimed is a powerful, courageous, and deeply personal guide that challenges the conventional narratives around mental health. My friend Dr. Azi masterfully blends her lived experiences with rigorous research, offering a holistic, empowering approach to healing. This book is a beacon of hope for anyone who has felt trapped by a diagnosis, showing that thriving is not only possible but within reach. Dr. Azi's insights on the mind-body connection, the importance of critical self-awareness, and the transformative power of lifestyle changes make this an essential read for those seeking to reclaim their mental well-being."

—Moshe Gersht,
Spiritual Teacher & WSJ Bestselling Author

Dr. Azi Jankovic guides and empowers us with authenticity drawn from her mental health history, coupled with extensive research, on how we can take greater control over our wellbeing with greater balance and positive change in our lives."

—Rabbi Elie Spitz,
Author of Healing from Despair: Choosing Wholeness in a Broken World

Mental Health, Reclaimed is a love letter and a lifeline to anyone who has felt misunderstood by the mental health system. It is a must-read for anyone navigating the complexities of mental health. I recommend this book to anyone ready to reclaim their health and discover the profound connection between nutrition, lifestyle, and mental well-being.

—Sheri Levy,
Board Certified Functional Diagnostic Nutrition Practitioner, Certified Holistic Health Practitioner, Nutrigenomics, Microbiome Specialist, SexyStrongLife

MENTAL HEALTH, RECLAIMED

A SIMPLE GUIDE TO THRIVING BEYOND LABELS OR LIMITS

BY DR. AZI JANKOVIC

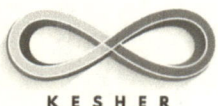

KESHER

ISBN
979-8-9986316-0-3   Softcover
979-8-9986316-2-7   Hardcover
979-8-9986316-1-0   eBook

This book is dedicated to every soul lost to broken systems. And to those still searching, struggling, or suffering, and wondering if there's another way.

May these pages be a light on your path.

CONTENTS

AUTHOR'S NOTE

On a chilly December morning in 2019, I received a phone call that shook me to my core. I was on a walk around the neighborhood, pushing my two-year-old son in the stroller, spending another day as a stay-at-home mom of four. Life was predictable: caring for the kids, simply getting through each day.

I picked up the phone, pausing the stroller to take in the view of the hills and fields in the distance.

On the other end of the line was one of my neighbors, a friend in her fifties who had always been a source of wisdom and advice. But this time, her voice carried something different—shock, devastation.

She told me that Gila (Hebrew for Joy), a teenage girl in a nearby community, had died by suicide the day before. No words can truly encapsulate the horror and heartbreak of hearing such tragic news. I felt gutted. A beautiful eighteen-year-old girl would never get the chance to grow up.

As she continued speaking, I realized that Gila had taken her own life in the psychiatric unit of a hospital I knew all too well. Instantly, my mind traveled back to the summer of 2018, when I had checked myself into that same psych unit, struggling with severe sleeplessness and manic, stress-related symptoms.

My mind instantly created a picture, a fantasy, which would never come to be. What if, two years earlier, Gila and I had crossed paths in that psychiatric hospital? She seemed like someone I would have befriended. When I saw her photograph for the first time, she immediately reminded me of my younger self.

Though I never had the chance to meet Gila, I did speak with her parents in the weeks that followed. They shared their story with me, opening up about the exhausting, heartbreaking struggle to find Gila the right help. They had fought tirelessly for her, and now, their pain was unimaginable.

*That conversation changed me. It solidified what I already knew deep down: **mental health must be at the forefront of our personal, family, and communal agendas.***

THE PROBLEM OF SECRECY AND MENTAL HEALTH

*For far too long, mental health has been shrouded in secrecy. But suffering in silence compounds the pain—it isolates people, preventing them from leveraging their networks for support, resources, and referrals. It leaves them at the mercy of a mental health system that doesn't always provide the answers they desperately need. And, according to the research, **there is a strong and consistent link between social isolation and levels of depression and suicide, not to mention elevated disease risks, impaired quality of life, and a significantly increased risk of early mortality.**[1]*

* * *

I know the struggle of keeping secrets intimately. For years, I navigated the maze of diagnoses, medications, therapies, and psychiatric hospitalizations—mostly in silence. I vacillated between hiding in bed when I wasn't well and keeping up with appearances when I could pull it off. Even my closest friends had no idea about my diagnosis. Looking back, I see just how much harder secrecy made everything.

*I've dealt with **severe** ups and downs since first being diagnosed with depression at 15 and then bipolar disorder at 17. I faced many of these challenges alone, fearing that if I were to share my experiences with others, I risked losing them. Today, I understand that keeping the challenging parts of my life a secret actually deprived me of the vital social support that could have been helpful in times of severe need.*

If I could go back in time and sit across from my fifteen or seventeen year old self, I am 100% confident that I could provide her with the tools and strategies to avoid 98% of the difficulties she endured. This is because I've been committed to ongoing learning throughout my struggle.

When I heard about Gila's tragic death on that chilly winter morning, I realized it was time to start speaking out. As an educator, I know the importance of role models in the learning process, and in the space of mental health, we need more of them—urgently.

And this is why I'm telling my story now. Because no one should have to struggle alone. Because there are answers. And because lives are at stake.

OUR STORIES MATTER

For a long time, I struggled to make sense of my own journey with mental health—how I got here, what went wrong, and what could have been different. Receiving that phone call in December of 2019 gave me the push to reflect, do the work, and come to terms with what I had been through. As much as I've accomplished in my life, it could have happened with so much more ease and flow if I had known then what I know now.

I have spent years unraveling my story, searching for patterns, and connecting the dots between my past and my present. I've come to understand that the mental health system—while sometimes helpful—failed me in ways I didn't always recognize at the time. I wasn't just a patient with symptoms; I was a person with a story that mattered, just like you and everyone else who is being reduced to a cluster of symptoms, aka – a diagnosis.

There was a time when I was a teenager in crisis, searching for answers. And then I went through a period of time as a young, overwhelmed working mom and doctoral student, plagued by perfectionism to the point of psychosis. And then years later, a post-partum spin-out, and several periods in between when symptoms of mania, depression, anxiety, and PTSD came creeping in, and I didn't know how to handle them.

It all started with a diagnosis—one that would set me on a path of learning, trial and error, and resilience. It's cliché to call it a journey—but that's what it was—one that involved years of research, personal struggle, and doing everything in my power to survive... and, ultimately, thrive.

It's taken me over twenty-eight years to get here.

For most of that time, I kept the details of my mental health struggles to myself, only sharing with immediate family. But something shifted as time passed, and I began to open up to friends. I realized that everyone I knew had been affected by mental health issues in some way—whether personally or through a loved one.

Then, in 2019, after I heard Gila's story, I made a decision.

While many people choose to keep mental health struggles private, this was no longer an option for me. I had seen too much, learned too much. Staying silent meant withholding hope, support, and guidance from those who needed it most.

Writing this book has taken time. I began in the spring of 2023 but had to pause when war broke out, shifting my focus to simply staying sane and functional. With G-d's help—and *the tools I'm going to share with you in this book—I not only managed to function, but I also learned how to thrive.*

Over the years, I've worked to put the puzzle pieces together. As I approach my 45th birthday, I can honestly say I've never felt better in my life. I believe there's a bigger picture to mental health than the disease model so many of us have been conditioned to accept. A diagnosis does not have to become a destiny. By understanding the factors that contribute to mental health challenges, we can learn to think beyond labels and step into new possibilities—realities free from debilitating symptoms and harmful side effects.

Far too many of us have been reduced to diagnoses that describe our symptoms—but overlook our souls. *We have been prescribed medications that blunt some of the symptoms but manufacture others. Stigmas that have positioned us as damaged, when in reality, the same society manufacturing those stigmas is what's damaged, captured, and corrupt on many levels.*

It's time for us to reclaim our power.

To step away from merely managing symptoms, and into identifying root causes and whole-person solutions.

To equip ourselves, one tool, one strategy, one fact at a time.

To move forward, one step at a time, toward true thriving.

Liberation begins with education.

A better way isn't just possible, it's within reach.

INTRODUCTION

"An abnormal reaction to an abnormal situation is normal behavior."

—Dr. Viktor E. Frankl,
Man's Search for Meaning

MY DIAGNOSIS

I was called to the stage to accept the annual Super-Star Writer of the Year Award at my high school graduation. It was June of 1998. I hobbled up to the stage on crutches to accept it. My left foot was in a cast and packed with metal screws from an amateur skateboarding accident earlier that spring. Even so, in that moment I felt on top of the world—recognized, celebrated, full of promise. What I didn't know was that everything I'd built was about to slip through my fingers.

Two weeks after graduation, after the cast had been removed, I boarded a plane to Europe and then Israel, unaware that the change in altitude would trigger a cascade of events—disrupting my sleep, my body, and eventually, my mind.

None of these details were relevant to the psychiatrist who diagnosed me in July of 1998. At age seventeen, I walked into his office for the first time. It was my first ever appointment with a psychiatrist. *Fifty minutes later, I walked out of his office with a diagnosis of a lifelong 'brain disorder.'*

That psychiatrist didn't ask about my injury or how experiencing foot pain on the airplane had pushed me into sleep deprivation. He didn't inquire as to my stress levels—he merely observed how I was acting within the confines of that fifty-minute appointment. And within the first fifteen of those fifty minutes, he had already assigned me a label that would largely define the next three decades of my life.

That moment changed so much.

By the end of that first appointment, I left with a diagnosis of Bipolar I and the understanding that I had a "genetic brain disorder," which would make me dependent on a strong chemical cocktail for the rest of my life. Unbeknownst to me in the moment, that same chemical cocktail would severely impair my functioning and make the simplest daily tasks feel nearly insurmountable.

The bipolar diagnosis threw me into a tailspin. My once-promising academic career crumbled—that upcoming fall, I lost a university scholarship because I could barely stay awake more than five hours a day. **Over the next twenty-five years, my life became a pendulum swing between having it all together (or at least appearing to) and crashing into a deep depression, mania, and even the psychiatric ward—seven times. Three of those psychiatric hospitalizations were against my will.**

As devastating and traumatizing as some of those experiences were, it was the shame around my secret that compounded the pain of it all.

For two decades, I kept my story a secret, believing that I would lose everything if anyone knew the truth about me.

BEFORE MY DIAGNOSIS

Up until the day of my bipolar diagnosis in the Summer of 1998, I had been a high achiever in school, creative, and involved in a number of extra curricular activities. In hindsight, however, there were warning signs for years that I was headed for a breakdown: I had been burning the candle at both ends in high school, working hard in school, and placing extreme pressure on myself to be a high achiever in all areas of my life. I was also "partying" on the weekends like most of the teens my age—engaging in high-risk behaviors that, while socially acceptable, were far from healthy for a developing brain. I had been dealing with symptoms of depression, trying to wash them away with a daily dose of Prozac that had been steadily increasing for over two years. I had been through traumatic events and didn't have the awareness or skills to process them properly. I had spent countless hours as a teen scouring the self-help shelves of Barnes & Noble for answers, a section in the bookstore that has since expanded and would be much more likely today to provide me with some answers.

The stigmas associated with mental health diagnoses in the 90s had influenced me to keep my situation a secret and push through while pretending to have my ducks in a pretty little line. Unfortunately, some parts of me needed help, and no one in the world, myself included, could see them. I managed to keep most of this under the radar until that summer of 1998, when my pain-induced sleeplessness landed me on the couch of my very first psychiatrist's office.

While there are some people who receive mental health diagnoses and respond well to conventional treatments, I was not one of these lucky few. Instead, I went on to suffer from side effects that left me nearly incapacitated. I went from being a straight-A student in high school with an academic university scholarship to failing out of my freshman year of college and seriously doubting if I'd ever achieve my dreams of living a full life or fulfilling my potential.

Fortunately, a small, still voice inside my heart moved me to question how this was remotely possible. My diagnosis had been slapped on hastily, without a single question about how nutrition, sleep, lifestyle, or past trauma **may have created the perfect storm that landed me on that psychiatrist's couch in the first place.**

OUR SHARED EXPERIENCE

Looking back now, I understand that my experience is far from unique. In fact, it's become alarmingly common. While every mental health journey is different, countless others have lived through disturbing parts of my story:

- We were diagnosed in under an hour, without any real examination of our lifestyle, nutrition, sleep habits, blood work, trauma history, or medical background.

- We were given pharmaceuticals with efficacy barely exceeding that of a placebo—or worse, medications with severe, lifelong side effects.

- We were never taught about lifestyle factors that can influence mental health, nor were we told how to use nutrition, movement, sleep, or stress management to prevent future episodes.

- We were told that depression, anxiety, and other mental health symptoms were simply to be expected in this modern era—and that with enough therapy, enough pills, and enough therapy bills, our symptoms *might* improve. At least a bit.

- We were never explicitly taught how to avoid manic, depressive, or anxious states, nor were we told that there are physiological, social, psychological, and spiritual pathways both into and out of these states.

At age 17, I didn't know how to question anything I was being told. I initially assumed psychiatry was based on cutting-edge science and that my diagnosis was as concrete as a blood test result. But over time, when this 'cutting-edge science' wasn't working, I began to do what I always did when faced with a challenge: I searched relentlessly for answers.

A LIFELONG SEARCH FOR THE TRUTH

I've been obsessed with self-help for as long as I can remember—ever since eighth grade when my dad handed me a copy of Dale Carnegie's *How to Win Friends and Influence People*. After my diagnosis, I practically moved into the self-help section of Barnes & Noble, scouring every book I could find for guidance on my situation.

Resources on mental health were much more limited in the 90s. **Conventional treatments were framed as the only viable path forward, and psychiatry's approach seemed set in stone: Diagnosis, medication, talk therapy, repeat.**

During those same years, my grandfather—a seasoned cardiologist who dedicated his life to medicine—was also perplexed by what I was going through. Until his passing in 2004, he often reflected on the tremendous progress made in nearly every other field of medicine, yet, much to his frustration, psychiatry had remained largely stagnant.

MENTAL HEALTH RESOURCES TODAY

Thankfully, the landscape has begun to shift, albeit slowly. We now have immediate access to an unprecedented wealth of information—insights that were once buried in research papers, inaccessible to the public, or outright dismissed by the conventional medicine establishment.

Some of these insights have come from groundbreaking research that challenges outdated assumptions. Others have emerged from a growing movement of educators—doctors, therapists, researchers, and healers—who bravely share what they've learned, even at the risk of being labeled "unconventional" or worse. Fortunately, many of these healers are far more committed to saving lives than caring about the name-calling.

It has taken a considerable amount of research, trial and error, and relentless searching to finally discover what truly works for me—what actually helped me break free from debilitating mental health symptoms once and for all.

If you've ever struggled with your mental health or watched a loved one suffer, you know how desperate and isolating it can feel.

THE RISE OF MENTAL ILLNESSES

The research is clear—in the year 2025, mental health challenges affect all of us, whether personally or through a significant relationship. Half the population alive today will be diagnosed with a mental health disorder.[2] If you don't personally fall into this statistic, chances are that you're closely connected to someone who does. Tragically, many suffer silently, burdened by shame and the false belief that they're broken, alone, and without hope. Unfortunately, this only makes the suffering more unbearable. **Mental health challenges have become so commonplace, and at the same time, so many people feel the need, and understandably so, to keep their challenges under wraps.**

Over the nearly three decades after my bipolar diagnosis, I did everything in my power to reclaim my mental health, defy my diagnosis, and live a full life. By the grace of God, with the help of countless dedicated human beings, and with the power of my inner teenage rebel, I have gone on to achieve many of my life goals and dreams.

THE OTHER SIDE OF THE HEALING PROCESS

After my initial bipolar diagnosis threw me off course, I was able to drop back into university, completing a bachelor's degree, teaching credential, a master's degree, and finally a doctorate. This year, I'm turning forty-five. I've been happily married for twenty-two years and have an incredible relationship with my husband and our four children. Ten years ago, our family fulfilled a dream of moving across the world and acclimating to a new country, new language, and a new culture that we cherish immensely. I've been blessed to engage in meaningful work across disciplines that light me up and make the world a better place.

While I'm incredibly grateful to be where I stand today, I also know that these accomplishments were *immensely* more difficult because I had to navigate serious mental health challenges without clear guidance about how to do so.

I'm blessed with deep, meaningful relationships with family and friends, work that I find truly fulfilling, and a spiritual philosophy that brings me a sense of peace—sometimes even bliss.

I've learned to embrace the full spectrum of my emotions, including the hard ones, as an essential part of being human. Today, I wake up with a sense of purpose I once thought was impossible.

It took a journey into darkness for me to finally find and embrace this light. Each day of this life feels like a gift, not only because I feel well enough to live it fully, but also because I've been on the other side. **I know what it feels like to be completely miserable—to genuinely wish I didn't exist and think the world would be better off without me.** The depth of that suffering has made the experience of wellness all the more vivid, and it's led me to a deep, abiding sense of gratitude.

If I had followed the advice of most of the mental health practitioners I encountered over the years, my life would look very different today. I say this with confidence because I've been there—unwell, trapped in misery, and caught in a relentless cycle of despair. I've hit rock bottom more times than I can count. I've faced moments so dark and chaotic that I truly wondered if I'd ever make it back. Yet, through all of it, I've learned and grown in ways that now allow me to offer hope and guidance to others walking their own difficult paths.

THE JOURNEY IS NOT LINEAR

If I had known then what I know now, I could have avoided significant hurdles along the way. Feeling better *could* have been so much simpler, but accumulating the knowledge and skills to navigate my complex wellness puzzle took three decades to piece together. The journey was not a straight line.

I spent several weeks of my life locked in six different psychiatric wards in two different countries. In those weeks, I often wondered if I'd ever regain my sanity or see the light of day again. I've also spent a cumulative total of two years in bed, barely functioning and almost totally incapacitated by medications and treatments that did not address the root cause of my suffering. Ultimately, I missed out on a lot of living and thriving because I was suffering from severe mental health challenges that nobody, including expert-level professionals, seemed to understand or be able to address fully.

While the journey has been incredibly painful at times, I consider myself lucky and blessed to have made it out the other side alive and quite well.

THRIVING IS POSSIBLE

If you or someone you care about has received a mental health diagnosis or is suffering from symptoms, you are now the *norm* and not the *exception*. For the lucky few, a conventional approach—perhaps a prescription and some talk therapy—may do the trick to get you back on your feet and feeling like yourself again. In the last three years since going public with my story, I've heard a handful of success stories sounding a lot like this. However, the majority of people who have confided in me haven't been so lucky or blessed, and I empathize because I know how difficult it can be to struggle without clear answers. I also empathize because living with anxiety, depression, addiction, and a whole slew of mental health symptoms has become a sign of our times. Everyone has a story when it comes to mental health.

THE SENSITIVE ECOSYSTEM OF THE HUMAN BODY

Over the years, I've often wondered, what are we missing that has led to this mental health epidemic? Mental health isn't just one slice of the pie—it's the plate holding everything together. Feeling well or unwell can make or break our entire lives. How can similar people, even twins, go through the same experience and have vastly different responses? The way we feel mentally and emotionally is the filter through which we experience our lives. Our minds are inextricably linked to our emotions through a complex physiology that is much more widely understood than it was in the 90s. The emotional state is interdependent on our thought patterns, social influences, culture, environment, and what our bodies do or don't metabolize.

As resilient and miraculous as the human body may be, it is also a sensitive ecosystem that can be thrown wildly out of balance by a myriad of influences. Yet, the experience of being diagnosed over the course of one short doctor's visit, and without analyzing those myriad influences, has become the norm. Prescriptions are being handed out at all-time high rates, while by and large, the mental health crisis continues to spiral out of control. I have the utmost respect for those who go into healing professions and believe that medical doctors must choose their profession to improve and save lives. Unfortunately, however, the medical systems in many places are not set up to do as much.

FINDING YOUR ROOT CAUSES

Ultimately, I have come to understand that there are root causes to many, if not all, mental health symptoms. **While this science is still evolving, the cutting edge of research in this space has identified the major building blocks of mental health.** It would be convenient if the solution could be bottled up and sold in pill form, but for better or worse, the situation is more complex than this for most people.

Mental health diagnoses are being handed out at an alarming rate across the modern world, often based on superficial, quick assessments of symptoms. These symptoms are then framed as incurable, lifelong disorders, with pharmaceuticals offered as the primary—if not sole—solution. What's missing from this approach is a thorough investigation of the *underlying root causes* of these symptoms. Today, we are at a pivotal moment when this information is available to us. Unlike thirty years ago, when the mental health crisis began to escalate, we now have far greater insight into the root causes of these challenges.

The good news, however, is that there are solutions, and many of them are right at our fingertips. Unlike in 1998, when the only sources of information were Encyclopedia Britannica and the self-help section of the local book store, we have a plethora of information available to us that can help us shed light on how, as a society, we got to such a dark place by way of mental health.

Over the past three decades, I've been on a relentless quest to uncover answers to four critical questions:

1. What are the underlying causes of our global mental health epidemic?

2. What solutions exist—free of harmful side effects—that aren't yet being widely promoted?

3. Is it possible to *prevent* future mental health struggles by taking a proactive approach?

4. How can someone with a mental health diagnosis move beyond merely surviving and unlock their potential to truly thrive?

The answers I've discovered have transformed my life—and I believe they can transform yours, too. In the following pages, you're going to learn about the latest research and an individualized approach to feeling better and thriving.

TAKING YOUR HEALTH INTO YOUR OWN HANDS

By the end of this book, you'll understand why there is no shame whatsoever in experiencing mental health symptoms. You'll discover the missing pieces of the greater mental health conversation, and you'll explore a path less traveled that transcends mere symptom management, guiding you to uncover root causes instead. You'll walk away with the knowledge, skills, and resources to better navigate the most commonly experienced mental health difficulties. While I've been diagnosed and dealt with Depression, Bipolar, PTSD, and Anxiety, much of the research I'll be sharing with you relates to a wider range of diagnoses and symptoms.

Your pathway to thriving is going to be as unique as your fingerprint. You'll learn about the "big four" building blocks of thriving: Physiological

Psychological, Spiritual, and Social influences. You'll gain insight into how your body, mind, and spirit process the reality in which you find yourself and discover new avenues for making adjustments or "Upgrades," in a way that is practical, sustainable, and, believe it or not, even *enjoyable*.

UPGRADING

An "upgrade" refers to any intentional intervention designed to help us reclaim our vital energy and step into greater levels of functioning. Rather than viewing an upgrade as fixing what's 'wrong,' you can think of upgrades as self-directed shifts—chosen, not prescribed.

An upgrade reframes the process of healing and growth as a conscious elevation; a shift toward alignment, vitality, and wholeness. Whether it's a mindset shift, a nutritional protocol, or a boundary we set, an upgrade is a purposeful step that supports our highest function and well-being.

A FALSE NARRATIVE

Mental health has become industrialized, packaged, and often sold as a one-size-fits-all solution. Many of us have learned a narrative that a mental health diagnosis is a permanent label—a life sentence or, at best, a prescription for mediocrity and struggle. I'm a firm believer that this narrative is false. A growing number of people, frustrated by limited options and doomsday diagnoses, have gone on to create beautiful lives through a myriad of "alternative" or "integrative" avenues. I am one of them.

I lost precious years of my life—and came close to losing everything— by getting caught in the trap of this narrow perspective. **But I'm here to tell you: reclaiming your mental health and thriving is not only possible but within reach. It takes the right knowledge, intentional strategies, and practical tools.** While we aren't seeing these solutions being advertised on billboards or packaged as quick fixes, they are grounded in real-world experience, rigorous research, and a healthy dose of common sense.

As the mental health industry has expanded, mental health challenges have skyrocketed worldwide.[3] We are witnessing all-time high rates of mental illness, and yet many people are too burdened by shame to seek treatment.[4] I also wonder if what holds some people back from seeking treatment is a fear of the conventional treatments and their potential side effects. From where I sit today, I can absolutely understand this line of thinking. We need better options at scale.

I used to believe my suffering was inevitable. That I was doomed to struggle for the rest of my life. I subscribed to the disease model of psychiatry, which framed me as a passive consumer, dependent on a system that positioned itself as the authority responsible for fixing me.

I no longer subscribe to that belief. Through lived experience and extensive research, I've come to see that this model not only fails to support my well-being—it often undermines it. I now believe we can reclaim our power, and rewrite the script.

If you've ever questioned whether a different way exists—whether there are other paths to healing beyond what you've been told—then this book is for you.

If you've ever suffered from mental health symptoms or witnessed someone suffering, you know how challenging this can be, and you are very much *not* alone.

If you're questioning whether healing and thriving are possible, I invite you to suspend doubt temporarily. You've already taken the powerful step of picking up this book and affirming your belief, or at least your curiosity, about what's possible. If you've ever felt hopeless, my deepest compassion goes out to you—I know just how painful and overwhelming this feeling can be.

Three years ago, I could barely string together a sentence. My mind was clouded with fear and dread, and I was so sedated by psych medications that thinking clearly felt impossible. Today, I feel better than ever before, and I attribute that to everything I've finally been fortunate enough to learn and implement since then. This shift didn't happen overnight. But it did happen, and it's possible for you too.

Human beings have an extraordinary ability to adapt, build resilience, and move forward, despite seemingly insurmountable challenges. If we met today, you might never guess the depths of despair I've faced—but I've been there. The good news is that I found hope and thriving, and I believe you can, too. My goal is to help you tap into your innate human strength and build a life where you can truly thrive.

PART I

PSYCHOLOGY

CHAPTER 1

GETTING STARTED

"Barn's burnt down --
now
I can see the moon."
—Masahide

If you're reading this book, chances are you—or someone you care about—have been searching for answers. I want you to know that I've been there, on and off, for nearly three decades. Whether you're just beginning to explore this topic or have been immersed in it for years, I hope that what you read here feels like a hand reaching out, offering empathy, clarity, evidence-based tools, and a path forward.

Let me be clear about this from the get-go: I am not a medical doctor. My doctorate is in education—a field that taught me how to think critically, ask hard questions, and engage with complex systems in search of deeper understanding. While I hold deep gratitude for modern medicine and the life-saving technologies it has made possible, my own experience—and the experiences of so many others—has shown me that when it comes to mental health, something has gone awry. We're relying on a system that too often pathologizes normal human experiences, overemphasizes medication, and overlooks the basic building blocks of our mental health.

Since 1998, I've sat across from dozens of therapists, psychiatrists, medical doctors, functional practitioners, and healers of all kinds. I've explored their methods, immersed myself in research, and interviewed world-renowned experts in a search for answers. No one person had the full solution—but taken together, their insights formed a tapestry that helped me piece together what I needed for healing, resilience, and peace.

During my eight years as a graduate student in education in the United States, not once was I assigned coursework focused on integrating mental health education into schools. My colleagues and I watched students struggle with mental health, and some of those students were tragically lost in the struggle. Meanwhile, many of us were quietly struggling too. We often questioned why our curricula required students to memorize the periodic table or the dates of obscure battles, yet it imparted nothing about human psychology, emotional health, or basic well-being.

When I graduated from my doctoral program in 2015, my dissertation chair, Dr. Alan Green, handed me my diploma and left me with two words: "Seek justice." Reflecting on my own experiences—and the crisis I see so many teens and adults silently navigating—I know that the most just thing I can do with everything I've lived and learned is to write it down and share it widely.

While I can't go back in time and hand this book to my 17-year-old self sitting across from her first psychiatrist, on the brink of what would become an unimaginable mental health crisis, I can share it with you. My hope is that it guides you toward greater clarity, function, and thriving—and that in doing so, every ounce of my struggle will serve a greater purpose.

A BIT ABOUT ME

I was born and raised in coastal Southern California, shaped by public schools, sunshine, and a deep curiosity about the human experience. As a teenager, I found myself drawn to big questions—about meaning, healing, and why some people seemed to thrive while others struggled. I once dreamed of becoming a rabbi and began college at a Jewish university but withdrew for mental health reasons—a turning point that reshaped my life's trajectory.

Eventually, I found my way to UCLA, where I studied sociology, psychology, and Jewish studies. I met my husband the week I graduated, and shortly after, we journeyed to Jerusalem for nine months to study ancient Jewish wisdom. We returned to Los Angeles in 2004, just before the birth of our first daughter. Over the years, I became an educator, earned a teaching credential, completed grad school, and built a family rooted in love, learning, and service.

In 2015, we moved to Israel to pursue a long-held dream—one that also fulfilled the unrealized dream of my husband's grandmother, a Holocaust survivor who never had the opportunity to make the journey herself.

Over the years, as I checked off many of the boxes on my bucket list—marriage, children, career, degrees, a spiritual life, and a home in Israel—there was an undercurrent of struggle I couldn't ignore. For years, I wrestled on and off with mental health challenges, trying to reconcile the life I had built with the emotional pain I often carried. It wasn't until my seventh psychiatric hospitalization in 2022 that the pieces finally began to fall into place. I started to see not only my own story more clearly, but also the broader patterns—and these realizations became the foundation of this book.

This book is the culmination of everything I've lived, studied, and witnessed. It's not a one-size-fits-all solution. It's about giving you what bigger systems often don't: **perspective, choice, and trust in your own inner wisdom.** I'm not anti-system. I'm pro-awareness and believe in engaging thoughtfully with the systems around us, rather than surrendering blindly to them.

My goal isn't to tell you what to do—it's to help you build discernment, offer the frameworks and knowledge that can empower you to trust yourself, and become your own most powerful advocate.

Throughout this book, I introduce tools to support whole-person healing—from understanding your physiology and exploring functional medicine to examining your thought patterns, strengthening your relationships, and connecting with purpose. This is the path I've walked to reclaim my mental health, and it's one I believe anyone can walk—with the right support.

I've experienced mental health systems in both the U.S. and Israel. In both, I encountered a tragic gap: care that is often inaccessible, unaffordable, or reduced to a checklist of symptoms and prescriptions. I've been told that depression is a Prozac deficiency, that Bipolar disorder is lifelong and unchangeable, and that symptom management—not healing—is the best I could hope for.

Spoiler alert: none of this is based on fact.

Thankfully, not all practitioners think this way. Along my journey, I also met exceptional healers—people who looked deeper, listened longer, and treated me as a whole person, not a broken one. Their approach wasn't grounded in fear or rigid frameworks—it was grounded in possibility.

That's what I hope to offer you.

I've dedicated my life to education, exploration, and helping others think critically and compassionately about their own lives. My research spans education, mental health, nutrition, spirituality, functional medicine, and beyond. My desperation over the years has pushed me to take a broad approach, and if there's one thing I've learned, it's this: no single person or protocol holds your answer. But you do have the power to discover what's right for you.

You are not broken, and you are not defined by a diagnosis. You are a complex, capable, and whole human being. And you deserve the clarity, as well as the care and community that supports your fullest healing.

This book is here to be your companion—rooted in the truth that reclaiming your mental health is possible when you have the right information and tools in hand.

HELPFUL NOTES AND DISCLAIMERS AS YOU READ

- **Tapering Off Medications:** If you are experiencing side effects of medications or are interested in exploring tapering, it's always advisable to do so with the help of a trustworthy and accredited professional. Your life may very well depend on it.

- **Disordered Eating:** As a content warning for sensitive readers, please note that throughout the book, I discuss eating habits, nutritional plans, the history of restrictive dieting, and other topics related to physical and mental well-being and the health care system. If you have or have had a history of disordered eating behaviors, please let a medical professional or registered dietitian guide you before making changes to your diet or eating patterns.

- **Professional Supervision for Rigorous Diet Plans:** In chapter 8, I outline how adjusting to a ketogenic diet was life-changing for me. Please note that a highly controlled nutritional plan or elimination diet can negatively affect your body and may not be right for everyone, especially if you have underlying health conditions or take certain medications. Seek guidance and supervision from a medical professional or registered dietitian to make sure the plan aligns with your age, medical history, lifestyle, and other factors.

- **Physical Limitations and Injuries:** In chapter 10, I mention that movement is not a luxury but a necessity. I believe most people, even those with physical injuries or limitations, are able to find some type of movement or modifications that work for them. But some may not. The contents of this chapter are based on personal experience, research, and observations throughout my years of mental health advocacy. I want to acknowledge that this will look different for all people. If you have a physical injury, limitation, or disability, consult a physical therapist, doctor, or other qualified specialist who can provide personalized guidance, and always remember to listen to your body and move at your own pace.

THE COMPLEX HOUSEPLANT

As you read the following chapters, I invite you to keep the following in mind: in many ways, you are like a complex houseplant. If you've ever planted a garden or cared for a houseplant, you know growing a thriving garden usually requires more than just the occasional watering. From the type of soil, material and size of the pot, to the lighting, temperature, humidity, water levels, and fertilizer, countless factors influence the health of even the "simplest" living thing.

Now, imagine your beloved plant isn't doing well—its leaves are sagging or discolored, a common frustration even for dedicated gardeners. Your first instinct might be to feed it a chemical compound to "fix" the problem. While this might help in some cases, if the lighting, water, or soil conditions are off, no amount of chemical intervention will make a lasting difference. For example, a shade plant placed in direct sun—or a sun-loving plant left in the shade—will struggle to survive, let alone thrive.

THE BIG FOUR INFLUENCES

Humans, much like houseplants, require the right inputs to flourish. These inputs fall into four main categories: **Physiological, Psychological, Social, and Spiritual.** We are complex beings, inhabiting intricate bodies and deeply connected to the social and spiritual worlds around us. These factors play a vital role in our mental health and overall well-being.

We now have evidence that nutrition plays a critical role in brain health, yet many medical schools still fail to provide future doctors with adequate nutrition education.[5] This leaves far too many people experiencing mental health challenges, labeled as disordered, and prescribed long-term medications, often without addressing or understanding the root cause of the problem.

We also have evidence that certain supplementation and exercise protocols can be as effective, and even more effective, long-term, than commonly prescribed pharmaceuticals for certain conditions.[6] These are but two basic examples of how addressing the needs of the whole person can offer comprehensive and sustainable solutions for mental health symptoms.

When we talk about addressing the "root" of the problem, for humans, this means taking a good and honest look at the big four influences. While the psychological component may feel like it's "inside" us, and social influences appear "outside" of us, the interplay of our human systems is closely connected.

Physiology refers to what's happening in our bodies, and therefore, "inputs" such as nutrition, sleep, movement, light, and others can be shifted to create harmony within our systems. The interconnectedness of human systems is profound. The vagus nerve, a key component of the parasympathetic nervous system, connects the brain to vital organs, regulating stress responses and fostering physiological calm.[7] This intricately tuned system doesn't function in isolation —our bodies and minds are deeply shaped by the people and environments around us.

Social interactions, while appearing "outside" us, can actually affect what's going on inside. They can promote feelings of connectedness that stimulate vagal activity, enhancing emotional well-being and physical health.[8] This is just one example of how our inner world is shaped by external forces—part of a larger puzzle involving the 'big four' systems that work together to influence our mental and emotional well-being.

HOW TO READ THIS BOOK

Learning about the big four influences and how they're all connected helps to prime the pump as you think about your mental well-being. Mental health isn't one-dimensional—it's shaped by a dynamic interplay of biological, psychological, social, and spiritual factors. To make this easier to remember, I refer to them as the 4Ps: **Physiology, Psychology, People, and Purpose.**

<u>Physiology</u> refers to what's happening in the body—our brain chemistry, gut health, sleep, nutrition, and more.

<u>Psychology</u> encompasses our thoughts, beliefs, emotional patterns, and perception of past/ present/ future experiences.

<u>People</u> speaks to the influence of our relationships—how connection, community, and support (or lack thereof) impact our well-being.

<u>Purpose</u> reflects the spiritual dimension, which I define broadly. Whether or not you consider yourself religious or spiritual, at the heart of this idea is a sense of meaning—a belief that we're not merely drifting through space by chance, but that each of us is here for a greater purpose, and capable of living in alignment with it.

The 4Ps offer a whole-person framework for understanding and reclaiming mental health. This book is divided into sections based on the 4Ps.

Before you go any further on your journey to thriving, it's important to recognize the work you're already doing. In a world where trusting your ability to heal is an act of courage and defiance, you have already taken the most powerful first step: having the hope, faith, or sheer rebelliousness that there will be a light at the end of this very dark tunnel. Let your courage and strength be the lens through which you read this book and reflect on your healing journey, one step at a time.

Remember that no matter how many qualifications or accolades a professional may have, no one can play God with your destiny, and no one has a crystal ball. No one can predict your future or define your potential. Your life is ultimately shaped by the choices *you* make.

I hope you'll commit, right now, to being your best advocate. You were born with the potential to thrive. Don't let anyone—or any system—convince you otherwise. Stand firmly in your power, speak up for your needs, and become the fiercest advocate for your own well-being.

Here are three helpful truths to keep in your back pocket as you read this book:

1. Healing isn't always a straight line.

While you may experience sustained, ongoing improvement, healing is a process of discovery, growth, and self-love, but it's not always linear. You are the hero of this story, moving forward at your pace, even if you take two steps forward and then one step back.

The path may not always be linear, but that's what makes it extraordinary. You're in the driver's seat, the CEO navigating your own forward trajectory.

2. Your diagnosis is not your destiny; your symptoms need not define your story.

If you're dealing with unwanted mental health symptoms or care about someone who is, I want you to hear this loud and clear: your diagnosis is *not* your destiny. You don't have to resign yourself to a lifetime of side effects, suffering, or mediocrity. Deep down, you may already sense that there's a better way—and I'm here to confirm that you're right.

3. Your progress is unique to you.

Healing isn't about fitting yourself into a rigid box of "healed" or "not healed." It's about recognizing that your journey toward greater well-being and thriving is uniquely yours. Only you can truly feel what progress looks and feels like, and only you can define what thriving means in your life. This requires tuning in to how you feel, which you may need to take some time with. **This is also an open invitation to get clear on how you want to feel and to envision the life you want to live. This is your permission to dream. I am a big believer that dreams can come true when we are clear not only about what we want but also why we want it.**

CALLING UPON HOPE

Hopelessness and doubt can act as *protective* and even *survival* mechanisms. While we humans are strong and resilient, we're also wired to conserve energy. If you believe the thought that you're beyond hope, you're also, perhaps unknowingly, giving yourself permission not to make an effort and to avoid the anguish of failure.

On the flip side, when you believe that healing is possible, this belief alone can initiate significant psychological changes. Research on the **placebo effect** shows that a belief in the possibility of improvement can activate real healing responses in the brain and body.[9]

Let me be clear: None of your mental health symptoms are your fault—they are signs and symptoms that the symphony of your systems is out of harmony. These imbalances have become a sign of our times.

Here's what I want you to know: the healing process we're about to embark on doesn't have to *feel* hard to be effective. It is not a prescriptive, all-or-nothing solution. You can implement it in parts and still find relief. So, setting aside any possible doubts, just for a moment, you're invited to lean into a new possibility:

- Consider that your healing journey may be pleasant, rewarding, and even joyful.

- Imagine a future where you no longer recognize parts of the person you are today—because you've progressed so immensely.

- Consider that the labels you've been given are surface-level descriptions of your symptoms, and beneath them lie unmet needs that, once addressed, can unlock your potential not just to feel better, but to truly thrive like never before.

THE POWER OF POSSIBILITY

This is the power of possibility, and you can access this power on your path to healing. I don't say this as someone speaking in theory, but as someone who is walking this road myself. Today, I'm standing in a place that I never thought possible. I have the roadmap that has guided me here, and in the following pages, I'll be walking you through each and every step. I intimately know the pain of hopelessness, but today I'm living proof that there is hope—and I believe you can have this too. Now that we've gotten acquainted, let's begin your journey to reclaim your mental health and THRIVE!

CHAPTER I SUMMARY

KEY CONCEPTS

1. **Healing requires a whole-person approach.** Mental health is influenced by four key areas, the 4Ps: physiology, psychology, social environment (people), and spirituality (purpose). Just as a plant requires the right soil, light, temperature, and water to thrive, humans need attention to these four areas to thrive.

2. **Healing is not a one-size-fits-all process.** Because we each have different needs, stressors, lifestyles, resources, etc., we each require a unique path to healing. Take your mental health into your own hands by being curious, researching, and experiencing for yourself.

QUESTIONS

1. What could it feel like to trade hopelessness for possibility? What beliefs or doubts might you gently release to make room for healing and growth?

2. If you truly believed that your symptoms or diagnosis didn't have to define your future, what hopes might begin to bloom? What would thriving look and feel like—for you?

3. Healing isn't a straight line—but an individualized, unfolding journey. How might this perspective shift the way you view your own path?

4. How might adopting a learning mindset support you in moving forward—especially when it comes to your healing, growth, and relating to the world around you?

CHAPTER 2

TOOLS TO STEP INTO HEALING

*"The wound is the place where
the Light enters you."*

—Rumi

When I was nineteen months old, I made a mistake that would haunt me for the rest of my life. I was lying on the Berber carpet of my grandparents' bedroom, watching my five-year-old brother pedaling on a white Tunturi stationary upright bicycle. Watching him ride that bicycle, moving the pedals swiftly in circular motions, I wanted nothing more than to join in the fun. I toddled over, stuck my foot in a pedal, and somehow, over the course of whatever transpired next, severely injured something in my right heel. The details of this event have become a bit fuzzy in my mind over the four decades since it happened, but what I do know quite clearly is that *I* wasn't the only one who made a massive mistake that day.

The other person who made a mistake was an adult, entrusted with my care. He was the radiologist in the emergency room who overlooked the fracture in my right heel bone. Weeks after I was sent home from that emergency room and told there was nothing wrong with my foot, a second medical doctor—my Grandfather of blessed memory, discovered that there was indeed a fracture. It had been missed in the ER, and now it was too late to fix the problem. My injury, combined with the improper reading of my X-ray, resulted in a lifetime of chronic foot pain and confusing messages about my identity and the possibility of trusting others with my care.

I came out of my foot injury traumatized, carrying with me an enduring belief—one that took root as early as nineteen months old—that I was somehow beyond help. While the adults around me puzzled over why I still wasn't walking, having been led to believe that "nothing was wrong" with my foot, I was trapped in a world of persistent, unexplained pain. Not only was I suffering physically, but I was also beginning to question who I could trust. What did it mean if everyone told me I was fine, but I didn't feel fine? Was something wrong with *me* for feeling pain? Was I weak? Abnormal? Or worse—did no one truly understand, and maybe no one ever would?

Looking back, one of the unexpected gifts of that experience—though it took years to recognize—was the inner strength it sparked. I learned to be stubborn, and even defiant when necessary, in the pursuit of real solutions. I learned to question authority, to trust my instincts, and to keep searching when something doesn't feel right—even if it means getting a second, third, or twentieth opinion. **While the foot injury initially led me to doubt myself, it also taught me something invaluable: no one can truly understand what I'm feeling or what I need unless *I* am clear about it—and willing to speak up with persistence and conviction to have my needs met.**

FROM VICTIM MENTALITY TO VICTOR MENTALITY

Decades later, I realized how my self-image was affected by that incident. I subconsciously internalized the idea that I couldn't trust myself or medical professionals to make great decisions.

This message is the double-edged sword of a *victim mentality*. It says: I am incapable, and no one can help me. It is the epitome of hopelessness and despair.

It took decades to undo this subconscious dialogue and realize that there was a tremendous gift in my early life experience.

One of the most crucial lessons I learned is that we all make mistakes—toddlers, parents, and even doctors. In fact, medical professionals read a significant number of body scans incorrectly every single day. Recent data notes that while the general day-to-day error rate in radiology practice is estimated at 4–5%, much higher rates have been reported in targeted studies focusing on specific conditions or imaging types.[10]

Now, remember that these errors are being made in analyzing images, a much more straightforward task than assessing a complex mental health picture involving multiple systems in the body and an endless number of subjectively reported symptoms. When it comes to diagnosing mental health issues, the situation can be quite complex. Even with the most caring practitioner – such as a medical doctor like my grandfather, who was devoted to providing the best possible care in his role as a physician - understanding our mental health landscape is not remotely as simple as carefully reading an X-ray.

CRITICAL INSIGHT

The big takeaway from this incident and the mental health debacle that followed is the importance of getting to know oneself, contextualizing our experiences, and connecting with deep intuition. I call this "CRITICAL INSIGHT."

Critical Insight is a broad awareness of the internal and external systems that shape human life. It's the recognition of the often hidden mechanisms and structures within these systems and an understanding of how they influence your thoughts, behaviors, and overall well-being. Critical Insight also goes beyond observation—it's about taking action, consciously navigating systems, and making intentional choices about how you engage with them. Critical Insight can also lead you to challenge or transform the systems themselves to create a better, more equitable reality for yourself and others.

INTUITIVE WISDOM

A vital step in developing Critical Insight is learning to tap into your intuition. Your intuition helps you sense when something about the systems you're operating within doesn't align with your values or well-being. It allows you to discern when to question, when to adapt, and when to stand up for change. Combining intellectual understanding with intuitive wisdom makes Critical Insight a powerful tool for living consciously and authentically. Critical insight has led me to question authority and tune in to that still, small voice reminding me of the uniquely human capacity for resilience and thriving.

Honing your Critical Insight means refusing to settle for mediocre care. It means breaking free from unnecessary limitations that have been placed on your life and well-being. This book is intended to guide you to tune in to the quiet inner voice. It's here to remind you that you aren't broken or damaged—you aren't destined for anything less than an amazing life.

STEPPING INTO YOUR POWER

Starting the next chapter of your life after receiving a diagnosis or experiencing symptoms can feel like waking up on an unfamiliar planet— one where you don't speak the language or understand the culture. In many ways, my own early experiences as a patient navigating the mental health system mirrored what it felt like to immigrate to a new country: unfamiliar, overwhelming, and challenging to find my footing.

When my family immigrated to Israel in 2015, navigating a new culture came with unexpected lessons, like one slightly ridiculous predicament involving our refrigerator. We purchased a familiar brand fridge with a built-in ice maker shortly after moving in. When the installation man arrived, he informed us that it wasn't possible to connect the fridge to our home's water supply, meaning: no ice maker for us. Annoyed but eager to adapt, we accepted his explanation, assuming it was just "how things worked" in our new country. Looking back, it seems silly, but at the time, we deferred to the installer's authority without question. We hauled heavy bags of ice from the grocery store to our home for nine years, rushing to prevent them from melting. With a family of six, the bags always seemed to run out before anyone had time to get more. It wasn't a major crisis, but it was definitely inconvenient. Then, one spring morning last year, our handyman came over to hang a kitchen shelf. On a whim, my husband asked if he knew how to connect the freezer to the main water line for ice. Within 15 minutes, it was done. I stood there, frozen—like an ice cube—half in embarrassment that the solution was so simple, and half in gratitude for something I'd never appreciated as much as I did in that moment.

Reflecting on this story through the lens of Critical Insight, there are a few valuable lessons to unpack. Nine years ago, the fridge installer had one job: deliver the fridge and plug it in. He likely had a packed schedule and no time for extras, like connecting an ice maker for an immigrant lady who could barely articulate her request in the local language. Fast forward nine years. We'd learned the language and built a relationship with a diligent handyman who took pride in his work. Paid by the hour and always eager to please, he had both the *time* and the *incentive* to solve our ice problem. It really was that simple.

TIME AND INCENTIVE

I'm sharing this somewhat embarrassing story to illustrate a parallel about "immigrating" into the mental health system. For many, the journey begins with a brief appointment with a general practitioner or psychiatrist, whose training often focuses on three things alone: assessing reported symptoms, assigning an "official" diagnosis, and prescribing a pharmaceutical solution to manage those symptoms.

While this approach may work for some, for others, it's like having your fridge plugged in but the ice maker left disconnected—functional in the most basic way, but far from optimal, and ultimately leading to unnecessary stress and hassles, to say the least.

Instead, imagine working with someone who goes beyond the surface, addressing all the underlying factors and ensuring everything is "connected." When that level of care is provided, the difference can be life-changing.

When it comes to our mental health, the stakes are much higher. We need to be vigilant about taking *radical personal responsibility* for our care.

YOU ARE THE CEO OF YOUR MENTAL HEALTH

The most important piece here is beginning to see yourself as empowered. Rather than seeing yourself as a patient, know that you are actually the CEO. The word **"patient"** comes from the Latin word **"Patiens,"** meaning **"one who suffers or endures."** Over time, it took on its modern meaning, referring to someone receiving care for illness or injury. Interestingly, the word also connects to the idea of being patient, reflecting the endurance required during treatment and recovery.

While patience can be a virtue, do you really want the process of waiting, enduring, and suffering to be a part of your identity? I'm guessing not. While your practitioners hopefully have more than their fair share of expertise and compassion and will support you on your healing journey, *you* are ultimately the CEO of your mental health.

Being the CEO of your mental health means that you're empowered to:

- Seek out more than one opinion, especially when it comes to making important decisions about your care.

- Ask questions about your diagnosis, symptoms, and available treatments, so that you understand their potential effects on your mind and body.

- Choose care providers who believe in your best possible outcome. Ideally, a practitioner will partner with you to support your highest potential and long-term well-being, helping you not just get by but truly thrive.

- Insist that any care provider prescribing you a medication or recommending a lifestyle change clearly explains the *how* and *why* behind it. Ask whether the treatment has been studied, who it's been tested on, and for how long—because your health deserves nothing less than informed, transparent care.

- Make sure you understand the potential side effects of any medication or lifestyle adaptation that's recommended to you. This is especially important when it comes to medications that may cause addiction or dependency. Be sure to ask: Are there alternatives with fewer side effects? How difficult is it to taper off this med, and what does a safe tapering protocol look like?

Remember, your practitioner works for you, and not the other way around. You are no longer the PATIENT. You are the CEO of your mental health and your future.

By understanding the big four influences on our mental health (Physiology, Psychology, People, and Purpose), we can create the conditions for true healing, lasting change, and a thriving life. This approach goes well beyond symptom management, creating transformation from the core. In a world where diagnoses are often made in minutes and medications—sometimes addictive or harmful—are prescribed without first exploring alternative paths to well-being, it's vital to approach healing with Critical Insight. This awareness can be the turning point between merely surviving and truly thriving.

By embracing Critical Insight, you take ownership of your healing journey, empowering yourself to chart a path toward greater health and a more fulfilling life. This is about:

- Taking radical personal responsibility

- Setting goals for yourself

- Overcoming fears

- Committing to healing

- Consistently putting one foot in front of the other with intention and awareness

In order to step into this path, you can answer some or all of the following reflection questions to get started:

REFLECTION QUESTIONS

TAKING RADICAL PERSONAL RESPONSIBILITY

- Have you been waiting for someone else to change things for you, and if yes, what would it look like for you to take responsibility for your progress instead?

- In which domains of your life can you ask for, or recruit more help and support? In which domains do you want to take more action on a personal level?

SETTING GOALS FOR YOURSELF

- What does thriving look like for you?If you could accomplish one meaningful shift in your mental or emotional well-being over the next three months, what would it be?

OVERCOMING FEARS

- What fears have been holding you back from making changes you know you could benefit from?What might become possible if you are to become driven not by fear, but by hope and faith in a positive outcome?

COMMITTING TO HEALING

- What does a true commitment to your healing look like—not just in theory, but in daily life?What practices or habits are you willing to try (or return to) in service of that commitment?

CONSISTENTLY PROGRESS WITH INTENTION AND AWARENESS

- What are some small, intentional steps you can take that align with your healing journey?

THE ECHO METHOD: A SIMPLE TOOL FOR THRIVING

One of the biggest lessons I've learned from years of therapy, countless self-help books, and even my time as an inpatient is that knowledge alone only takes you so far—it's what you *integrate* into your daily life that creates sustainable well-being.

The challenge is that integration requires change, and change can often feel uncomfortable or overwhelming. To address this challenge, and to make the process of upgrading your life both realistic and enjoyable, I'd like to introduce you to the *ECHO Method*—a simple, four-step framework rooted in research on habit formation. This method has been my anchor for creating lasting change and thriving, and it's designed to guide you through your journey incrementally.

Think of the ECHO Method as your personalized companion along the wellness journey. It's an adaptable approach that's worked wonders for me, and I believe it can work for you, too. To take charge of your healing process, adopting a scientific approach is essential—testing one variable at a time, observing the results, and refining your strategy to discover what works best for you.

Some of the upgrades I'll be recommending later in the book are relatively simple, like spending 15 minutes in the morning sunlight or practicing intentional deep breathing. Others, such as crafting a personalized nutrition and movement plan, require more effort but can yield profound rewards. The ECHO method can guide you in making these practices manageable. Here's how it works:

E: EDUCATION

Educate yourself with the information available. Explore and understand lifestyle adaptations that can serve as personalized upgrades to support your well-being by learning the "how" and "why" behind each upgrade. You become an active participant in your wellness journey, empowering yourself to choose what aligns with your unique needs and circumstances. Arm yourself with the relevant facts, concepts, procedures, beliefs, and strategies needed to test out a new variable on your healing journey.

C: CURIOSITY

Curiosity is having an open mind and heart. It's the willingness to remain open to the possibility of change, growth, and healing—even if it feels out of reach. It's a mindset of exploration that allows you to step outside your comfort zone to try new approaches. By cultivating curiosity, you allow yourself to imagine outcomes beyond what you previously believed possible. At any moment, you can ask yourself, *"What could my life look like if this intervention works for me?"* as well as "What might this feel like," and "What if it won't be as difficult as it seems?" These questions can spark the motivation to take meaningful steps toward transformation.

H: HEALING

The Healing process happens on its own timeline. This is where the magic happens—taking action to implement what you've learned and observed. Some interventions bring about almost immediate benefits, while others may take more time. This healing stage is all about *feeling and experiencing* each element of the healing process: staying aware, mindful, and getting in touch with the details of your experience.

O: OBSERVATION

The observation stage is when you step away and take a bird's-eye view of your process, reflecting with your mind and body on how each intervention is impacting your functioning. With this mindful perspective, you can decide whether to continue, tweak, or replace each intervention to align with what your mind, body, and soul need.

You are a unique, one-of-a-kind being, made up of trillions of cells working in near-perfect harmony. While practitioners and experts can offer invaluable guidance and support, only you can accurately understand your body and mind by experiencing it from the inside out. Healing is not about one-size-fits-all solutions; it's about discovering and co-creating the unique recipe that will serve you.

The beauty of the ECHO Method is that it's always with you—ready to guide you, no matter where you are on your journey. Whether an adaptation becomes an upgrade that you decide to integrate or let go of, there's no such thing as failure in this process. There is only feedback.

We all want to feel better, and it's truly rewarding when something works and becomes a transformative part of your life! But even when something doesn't quite fit, that's still a valuable discovery. Don't despair if you need to pivot – this is still progress. Knowing what *doesn't* work for you is crucial to understanding your needs and fine-tuning your path. The key is to remain hopeful, curious, and committed to learning and growing with the ECHO Method as your guide.

The ECHO Method is not a prescription; it's a process to guide you to step into your role as the hero of your healing journey. Healing and thriving are lifelong journeys, inviting you to experiment, observe, and refine your methods. Over time, you'll uncover your personalized formula for wellness, and you can continue using the ECHO method as you heal to greater and greater levels of well-being. No one can do this process *for* you. Only you can get 100% in touch with your personal experience.

RECLAIM YOUR POWER

For many, receiving a diagnosis can be life-altering. I know this feeling firsthand since the day I received a bipolar diagnosis and was turned into someone I no longer recognized. No matter the severity of your situation, the process we're embarking on is one of reclaiming your power, prioritizing your ability to thrive, and understanding that as you step into your true potential, not only do you transform your own life, but you also contribute to building a stronger, more whole world.

CHAPTER 2 SUMMARY

KEY CONCEPTS

1. **Critical Insight is a profound awareness of the internal and external systems that shape human life.** It's the awareness of the often hidden mechanisms and structures within these systems and the understanding of how they influence your functioning and overall well-being.

2. **Even experts make mistakes.** Sometimes, even doctors and professionals make errors, particularly in fields like mental health, where diagnoses are made subjectively. Recognize the *strengths and limitations* of systems designed to help while making informed decisions in the process.

3. **You are the CEO of your mental health.** Rather than viewing yourself as a passive "patient," see yourself as the CEO who can take control of your well-being, seek second opinions, ask questions, and make decisions that align with your needs and values.

4. **The ECHO method illustrates how healing isn't about one-size-fits-all solutions.** It's about experimenting, observing, and refining your approach. The ECHO Method

(Education, Curiosity, Healing, and Observation) is a structured process for making upgrades.

QUESTIONS

1. Using the Curiosity approach in the method, what might sustainable healing look like for you?

2. What would it look like for you to step into being the CEO of your mental health? How could leaning into this identity empower you to take charge of your future?

3. How might certain beliefs be impeding your progress? What new belief could you adopt to support your ongoing growth and improved functioning?

4. Healing begins when we connect deeply with our own story. If you were to tell the truth of your mental health journey—just for you, without filters or outside expectations—what would it sound like? What have you survived, discovered, and learned so far along the way, and what do you hope to learn and achieve moving forward?

MEDICATIONS: A NUANCED APPROACH

"For years, I'd been classified as treatment resistant, but a spark had ignited in me: it was time to resist treatment."

—Laura Delano, *Unshrunk*

In the late 1990s, most visits to a psychiatrist were shrouded in secrecy, wrapped in shame and stigma. My first appointment with Dr. Grimsky (pseudonym) in July of 1998 was no exception. Walking into the waiting room, I flipped a light switch on the wall to alert the psychiatrist that we had arrived. Patients in this office would enter and exit from two different doors to ensure that one patient would not see the other. This setup is not uncommon in therapy and psychiatry clinics to ensure patient privacy. While there may be some value in this, we can also understand how the interest in this high level of privacy points to a demand in keeping psychiatry and therapy visits, well... private, and perhaps even secret.

I sat in Dr. Grimsky's waiting room—a formal, wood-paneled room with dark green drapes covering the window—clutching a sliver of hope that he'd prescribe me some pills to help me sleep, and I'd move on with my life feeling refreshed. Certainly, modern medicine could provide me with this, right? Even in my despair and confusion, after days of pain-induced sleeplessness, I imagined myself bouncing back resiliently over the course of the next few weeks and entering university like nothing ever happened.

Instead of having my hopes fulfilled, that visit to Dr. Grimsky became a defining moment, catapulting me into many months of serious dysfunction like nothing I'd ever experienced before. It was a meeting that would leave me grappling with a severe mental health diagnosis and the crushing belief that I was "incurable," "mentally ill for life," and had a "brain disorder."

After recounting the sleepless chaos of my recent days—pain from my injured foot on the international flights, hobbling down cobblestone streets in Rome, and hallucinating a spectrum of colors bouncing off the white stone walls in Jerusalem, Dr. Grimsky dismissed the foot pain part of my story as irrelevant. He swiftly diagnosed me with bipolar disorder, explaining that my sleepless circumstance was merely a coincidence, and that the bipolar symptoms would have somehow appeared even if I hadn't taken the trip.

I remember distinctly sensing that something was off in his assessment. Even so, I brushed off my instinct, telling myself that he was the one with the medical degree, and I was a mere high school graduate.

Looking back, I see him in the same light as the fridge installation guy who couldn't, or didn't want to, hook up an ice maker. This psychiatrist did the absolute bare minimum, scribbling out a prescription for Lithium in stereotypically sloppy handwriting. He declared my condition both lifelong and incurable.

Today, we have expert psychiatrists explaining how bipolar and other mental health-related symptoms can be caused by light sensitivity, stress, sleep disruptions, hormonal imbalances, street drugs, and even prescription pills, including SSRIs such as Prozac.[11][12][13]

But back then, the evaluation I received was reductive and devoid of nuance, slapping my parents with a $300 bill (much more in today's dollars) and leaving me stranded without understanding of how or why my sleeplessness had spiraled into symptoms of mania or what to do about it. I was prescribed Lithium and several other medications, which, much to my chagrin, only compounded my suffering.

PSYCH MEDS: A DOUBLE-EDGED SWORD

The adverse effects I experienced are a clear example of *iatrogenic harm*—
health complications caused not by illness, but by the treatment itself. In
psychiatry, this often shows up as medication side effects, withdrawal
symptoms, or emotional and cognitive distress brought on by the very
interventions meant to help. My journey revealed firsthand how psychiatric
treatments, even if well-intentioned, can sometimes create more profound
suffering and new health challenges instead of healing.

LITHIUM

Lithium has been hailed by some in the medical field as the gold standard
for managing bipolar disorder. Its therapeutic effects are believed to involve
modulation of neurotransmitter systems, including dopamine, glutamate,
and GABA, as well as alterations in sodium transport across cell membranes.
The same 2024 study that hails Lithium as a gold standard treatment also
posits that, "it has been very difficult to identify the key mechanism of action
of Lithium in regulating mood."[14] For many people, Lithium can also have
difficult and even unbearable effects, which may be why its use has declined
consistently for decades. I know just how miserable these effects can be.

Dr. Joanna Moncrieff is a British psychiatrist and academic renowned
for her critical perspective on mainstream psychiatric practices, particularly
the use of psychotropic medications. She is a Professor of Critical and
Social Psychiatry at University College London (UCL) and a consultant
psychiatrist within the National Health Service (NHS) in London.

As a leading figure in the critical psychiatry movement, Dr. Moncreiff
offers a vital perspective on the use of Lithium in treating bipolar disorder.
She challenges the conventional view of Lithium as a "gold standard"
mood stabilizer, arguing that its therapeutic effects are not well-understood
and may be more attributable to its general sedative properties than to
specific mood-regulating mechanisms.

In her article *"Reasons Not to Believe in Lithium,"* Moncrieff explains
that Lithium is a neurotoxin that inhibits nervous system functioning,
leading to feelings of drowsiness and lethargy. She explains that these
effects were initially observed in animal studies and later in humans,
suggesting that Lithium's sedating effects may stem from its overall
dampening of neural activity rather than targeted mood stabilization.[15]

In 1998, I hoped Lithium would be my salvation, but instead, it plunged me into a fog of exhaustion and numbness so thick I began to feel like a completely different person. By the time I started college, I was sleeping up to 20 hours a day, unable to stay awake in class or muster the energy to engage in daily life of any sort. My hunger was insatiable, my body heavy and lethargic. I gained over 20 pounds in a matter of weeks, and a cold, dark cloud of daily despair replaced the vibrancy of my previous life.

I'd experienced depression before, but this was another level. The medication-induced numbness robbed me of even the smallest joys or pleasures. Food lost its flavor, music lost its charm, and the light at the end of the tunnel disappeared entirely. Basic socializing felt laborious, and my normal experience of empathy and connection with another person while in conversation was completely gone. I withdrew from university with failing grades and sadly had to move back home with my parents. My state of hopelessness and despair felt inescapable.

Around the same time that I withdrew from school, I also secretly flushed my medications down the toilet. I had no clue at the time how dangerous this could have been. For me, at age eighteen in the year 1998, it felt like my only option. Today, awareness around the downsides and dangers of medication is growing, and there is a growing body of board-certified psychiatrists who specialize in safely tapering off meds.

THE NUANCE OF MEDICATION

My experience with Lithium was extreme, but it taught me an important lesson: medication is nuanced, and it affects different people differently. You can find research on all sides of the pharmaceutical debate. Conventional medicine largely purports that meds are necessary for many, many diagnoses.

At the same time, a growing body of medical professionals is looking for root causes and focusing on a range of solutions, such as those included in this book. This growing group of practitioners takes a thoughtfully nuanced approach to medicine, and many are active in sharing their insights and research publicly.

In general, medical doctors who are certified in *functional medicine and integrative medicine* or who take a *whole-person* or *holistic* approach tend to look at the bigger picture in psychiatry because they are trained to look for root causes.

Functional medicine is a systems-based, patient-centered approach to health care that seeks to identify and address the root causes of illness rather than simply managing symptoms. It blends conventional medicine with evidence-based alternative practices and strongly emphasizes lifestyle factors such as nutrition, sleep, stress, relationships, and movement.

Instead of asking, "What drug matches the disease?" Functional medicine asks, *"Why is this symptom occurring in the first place, and how can we restore balance to the system?"*

Integrative medicine is a healing-oriented approach that combines conventional Western medical practices with complementary therapies, such as acupuncture, meditation, massage, yoga, or herbal medicine. It emphasizes the therapeutic relationship between practitioner and patient and treats the whole person: body, mind, and spirit.

Integrative medicine is often used in chronic disease management, cancer support, mental health care, and preventive health.

Medical doctors (MDs or DOs), nurse practitioners, and other licensed health professionals can pursue specialized training in these areas.

Functional Medicine Certification is often obtained through institutions like the Institute for Functional Medicine (IFM), which offers a rigorous certification program involving coursework, case studies, exams, and clinical practicums.

Integrative Medicine Certification is available through programs like the Andrew Weil Center for Integrative Medicine, which offers fellowships and board certification via the **American Board of Integrative Medicine (ABOIM)**.

Health coaches can also be certified in functional or integrative approaches, often through programs like the Functional Medicine Coaching Academy, which partners with IFM.

You can learn more about these approaches through organizations such as the Institute for Functional Medicine, the Andrew Weil Center for Integrative Medicine, the Cleveland Clinic Center for Functional Medicine, and the National Center for Complementary and Integrative Health (NCCIH). I have no affiliations with these institutions, but I do find their contribution to mental health and well-being quite important.

The functional medicine approach has gained popularity for its personalized, root-cause-focused model of care—but it is not without criticisms. One of the most significant critiques of functional medicine is that it can sometimes be **prohibitively expensive** for most people. Functional medicine practitioners often:

Spend more time with patients (initial visits may be 60–90 minutes or longer).

Order a wide array of **advanced lab tests**—including genetic, microbiome, hormonal, and toxin screenings—which can cost hundreds or thousands of dollars and are **typically not covered by insurance**.

Recommend **supplement regimens, personalized diets, or alternative therapies** that add to the out-of-pocket cost.

As a result, this model is often accessible only to those with higher incomes, leading critics to call it **"elite wellness"** or "concierge care." My goal in sharing what I've learned in the functional medicine space is to explain these health interventions in the simplest, most accessible way possible. I've also managed to make tremendous progress with relatively few functional medicine visits and out of pocket costs over the years, thanks to the honest and ethical functional practitioners I've been blessed to find and work with.

While the field of functional medicine may seem complex or out of reach, I believe that everyone deserves access to basic, empowering information about how the body and mind work together.

This book is structured to offer practical tools and insights that anyone can understand and apply—no expensive tests, complicated protocols, or medical degrees required.

I will also say that while working with the right functional or integrative practitioner may be more costly than going conventional in the beginning, if you are guided to adopt sustainable protocols, over time, you may benefit from saving time, feeling better, and even spending less money over the long-term on your medical care. As with every recommendation I'm making, this is a personal decision that you, as the CEO of your health, can make an informed decision about.

BENEFITS AND LIMITATIONS OF MEDICATION

For some people, medication may be a lifeline; for others, it can be a prison. Most of my best years since 1998 have been medication-free or nearly medication free, and there have also been periods when one pharmaceutical or another provided me with a specific benefit. The key is working with a medical professional who understands both the benefits and limitations of medication—and who is also open to exploring non-pharmaceutical interventions.

Medications are often heavily marketed, while natural, lifestyle-based solutions to management or treatment, like optimizing sleep or eating more nutrient-dense foods, are not directly connected to big industry and won't be promoted to you in flashy TV commercials or magazine spreads.

I believe healing can happen when we return to the foundational basics of looking after our physiology. For decades, societies have marketed packaged and processed foods as a form of liberation from the kitchen—prioritizing convenience over true care. But reclaiming our power means questioning these narratives and remembering that nourishing ourselves is not a burden, but a profound act of self-respect and resilience.

CRITICAL INSIGHT WITH MEDICATIONS

Maintaining a Critical Insight when faced with a prescription for medication is important. If you're being shown a potential solution, ask yourself the following questions.

1. Who is benefiting from selling you this thing?

2. Who benefits if you take it?

3. What could be the potential upside of taking this medication?

4. What could be the potential downside?

5. Are there free or inexpensive and sustainable alternatives not being directly marketed to you that may be helpful in your situation?

Today, more than 64% of American adults have taken prescription medication in the past 12 months.[16] Even more, 25% of US adults report taking four or *more* prescription medications regularly.[17] This is representative of a growing trend; psychiatric prescriptions are increasingly common as mental health diagnoses skyrocket. The number of patients diagnosed with mental health conditions increased by 39.8% between 2019 and 2023, rising from 13.5% to 18.9% of all medical patients during that period.[18] In the US and New Zealand, people are bombarded with direct-to-consumer advertising from powerful pharmaceutical companies, promising relief and solutions in slick, seductive commercial campaigns.

When it comes to medications, there is no one-size-fits-all, black-and-white solution for most cases. Psych meds can provide relief for some, particularly those experiencing severe and debilitating symptoms. For this group, the short term benefits may outweigh the drawbacks, and the right medication can be life-changing. At the same time, we need to consider the big picture around pharmaceuticals, especially in countries where for-profit companies own medications and insurance, such as in my birth country, the United States.

MASS OUTRAGE OF THE AMERICAN PUBLIC

The CEO of UnitedHealthcare, Brian Thompson, was tragically assassinated on December 4, 2024. He was fatally shot outside the New York Hilton Midtown hotel in Manhattan while attending an investors' conference. The motive was outrage, indicative of the mass outrage in the American public against the healthcare industry. While violence is *never* the answer, we see a swath of people across younger generations expressing clear support for the assassination, reflecting a deep frustration with the system. What is all this outrage about?

Let's pull back the curtain and have a look at what's happening in the for-profit American health insurance system. Chronic diseases are the leading causes of death and disability in the U.S., and they are also the primary drivers of the nation's $4.1 trillion in annual health care costs.[19] Mental health is deeply intertwined with chronic disease, both as a **contributing factor** and as a **consequence** of physical illness.[20] Mental health conditions, such as depression, can increase the risk of chronic diseases, and chronic diseases can, in turn, increase the risk of mental health conditions.

Medical care was patient-focused before the 1980s; doctors would visit patients in their homes and look at their family dynamics, environment, and lifestyle. (Remember our house plant analogy of whole-person health?) Those doctors spent time understanding the context of the whole person they were dealing with. My grandfather was one of those doctors who made home visits in that era. But in the 80s, insurance shifted to a profit-driven model, which we refer to as the Health Maintenance Organization (HMO).[21] This has undermined quality healthcare.

Not only did health insurance providers become profit-driven, but they also swallowed up Pharmacy Benefit Managers (PBMs), organizations whose original role was to keep the cost of pharmaceuticals down and ensure consumer affordability. The Federal Trade Commission (FTC) has found that major pharmacy benefit managers (PBMs), such as those owned by Cigna, CVS Health, and UnitedHealth Group, have been increasing drug costs instead of controlling them. The FTC's investigation revealed that these PBMs overcharged for medications, including cancer treatments, and engaged in practices that raised expenses for both employers and patients.[22]

The insurance companies are thereby incentivized to prioritize keeping patients on prescription drugs to generate recurring revenue, over providing preventative measures or costly surgical interventions. This is the monetization of chronic illness, and **mental health diagnoses are no exception to what's taking place by and large.** To understand why there is minimal focus on root causes like nutrition and lifestyle, we need to keep in mind *who* is benefiting from *what*.

CORRUPTION IN THE HEALTHCARE INDUSTRY

While this definitely doesn't apply in every country, corruption in the healthcare industry and in the government regulating bodies is not hard to uncover in the U.S. In recent years, we have evidence of FDA officials allowing highly addictive and deadly prescriptions onto the market with zero warning to the consumer, and months later transferring to high-paying roles in the very pharmaceutical companies that they had approved, lying blatantly to the public instead of ensuring proper safety regulatory measures.

The most infamous case is known as the Purdue Pharma scandal, which involved the unethical approval and aggressive marketing of OxyContin, an opioid eight times more addictive than hydrocodone. The FDA, under the leadership of Curtis Wright, who later joined Purdue, granted the drug a misleading label claiming it was less addictive and less prone to abuse, despite no human safety studies supporting these claims. This deceit contributed to the opioid crisis, which has claimed over 645,000 lives in the U.S., making it a stark example of profit-driven corruption at the expense of public health. The number of lives lost in this crisis surpasses the combined total of American deaths in World War I, World War II, and the Vietnam War. It's equivalent to the entire population of the city of Boston, Massachusetts, being wiped out, illustrating a catastrophic toll akin to a mass disaster occurring over decades, fueled by corporate greed and systemic failures.[23] The story has since been turned into a book as well as a full-feature Netflix series called "Painkiller."[24]

Healthcare companies drive systemic issues with pharmaceutical dependency and addiction, including the case of opioids. Healthcare costs are now the #1 leading cost of bankruptcy in the U.S, with federal budgets and employers strained by these rising expenses.[25] The ultimate cost, however, is paid in human lives, as systemic failures are causing addiction, despair, and unconscionable numbers of preventable deaths.

I highlight the systemic challenges we see today not to instill fear or outrage, but to emphasize the importance of acknowledging systemic issues in order to reclaim our mental well-being. Recognizing that we operate within imperfect systems can be empowering—it equips us with the insight to take ownership of our health, focus on what we can influence, avoid being victimized, and become agents of meaningful change in our own lives.

HEALTHCARE ENTREPRENEUR
TURNED ADVOCATE

Brigham Buhler is a healthcare entrepreneur and former medical device and pharmaceutical representative. While still in high school, his brother had an ACL injury, underwent surgery, and subsequently became addicted to his prescription opioids. Since his brother's death, Buhler has become an outspoken critic of the healthcare industry, sharing evidence around the corruption of insurance companies and the resultant devastating toll on human life.

He explains a few important facts. Namely, U.S. pharmacists are legally mandated not to inform the consumer about the availability of non-addictive alternatives or even the fact that their prescription may be available at a lower cost if they were to pay cash and *not* use their insurance "benefits" to buy the drug.[26] He has also been extremely outspoken about how many societal problems can be traced to problems in the drug industry.

While drugs classified to address mental health-related symptoms differ from opioids in their intended purpose, it's important to remember that all of these drugs are circulating through the same systems.

The field of psychiatry is far from immune to corruption. Its credibility has been declining in recent years, with experts coming out as whistleblowers revealing corruption, including leaders and prominent academics having alleged close ties to the pharmaceutical industry.

Like the Purdue case, we have evidence that academics and leaders in the field of psychiatry have publicly disregarded severe and even debilitating side effects of psychotropic drugs. The APA (American Psychiatric Association) has even admitted, albeit under pressure, "that over one third of its funding came from the drug industry."[27] We also have evidence that approximately *"60% of physicians who had served as panelists or task force members of the fifth edition of the American Psychiatric Association's Diagnostic and Statistical Manual of Mental Disorders received payments from industry... (totalling) $14.2 million... to 55 physicians with disclosures on the Open Payments database of the Centers for Medicare and Medicaid Services."*[28] This problem is particularly pervasive in the space of mental health, where meds are often a first line of treatment, and where patients are keeping their experiences private out of shame. The bottom line is that while ideally we would able to trust experts, that level of trust has been jeopardized by too many in the field and for far too long.

This is why now, more than ever, it's essential to become informed, ask questions, and take an active role in your own healing—because reclaiming your mental health begins with reclaiming your power to think for yourself.

DIAGNOSTIC INFLATION

There's another important issue to keep in mind when it comes to diagnoses in the latest version of the official Diagnostic and Statistical Manual of Mental Disorders (DSM-V) published by the American Psychiatric Association (APA). This is the "official" handbook used by clinicians to label mental health conditions Dr. Allen Frances, who was the former chairperson of the previous version (the DSM-IV) has a lot to say on the topic. While he's not completely writing off the field of psychiatry, he does call out some grave errors of its last few decades.

Dr. Frances notes that, "rates of Attention Deficit Disorder have tripled, and rates of Autism and childhood Bipolar Disorder have multiplied an incredible 40 times."[29] He points to the latest version of the DSM as having inflated these diagnosis rates. **The manual "...fostered an increasing tendency to chalk up life's difficulties to mental illness and then treat them with psychiatric drugs."**[30] Remember that these words are being spoken by *the* expert psychiatrist who was in charge of supervising the previous version of the DSM.

Dr. Frances' main concern with the current version of the DSM (DSM-V) is *diagnostic inflation,* again, the tendency to equate life's difficulty with a mental health diagnosis and treat it with drugs: pathologizing and medicating normal human behavior.

While Frances doesn't discredit every diagnosis, he's issuing a serious warning to the public that we need to be much more discerning about what we're diagnosing and medicating, especially because so many meds come with unwanted, unpleasant, and even extremely dangerous side effects. **Dr. Frances also urges medical experts to only diagnose after several sessions, sometimes even after many months, which is clearly not happening in most cases right now, according to the data.**[31]

THE OVERPRESCRIPTION PROBLEM

Mental health struggles can leave people feeling vulnerable. Feeling depleted and desperate, we turn to professionals for answers. Recent 2024 data indicates that "More than 60% of psychotropic medications were prescribed by providers other than psychiatrists (33.5%) or psychologists (2.2%), such as general practitioners, nurse practitioners, and physician assistants."[32] While the prescribers may be well-intentioned, many of these prescriptions address symptoms without ever addressing the more complex root causes of mental health symptoms.

In my own journey, I've been prescribed over 15 different medications for various mental health symptoms. A few have offered temporary relief, while most have worsened my situation. With all of this being said, I understand that there are instances in which medications may be medically necessary, helpful, and even life-saving.

To summarize my approach, I would choose the path of least harm, a "harm reduction" approach.

A harm-reduction approach to medication means meeting people where they are, without judgment, and offering support that prioritizes safety, choice, and empowerment. It's not about being "for" or "against" medication—it's about respecting an individual person's unique journey and providing the education and tools they need to make informed decisions. This approach emphasizes collaboration, personalized care, and minimizing risk, whether someone chooses to stay on medication, safely taper off, or explore alternatives. It recognizes that healing isn't one-size-fits-all, and that with the right support, people can reclaim agency and move toward true well-being on their own terms.

A GROWING MOVEMENT OF ALTERNATIVE SOLUTIONS

Research confirms that my experience with meds is not uncommon, and the movement around alternatives is growing. I'd like to highlight a few outspoken advocates for progress.

The medical doctors who specialize in psychiatry, whom I have come to respect the most, highlight the need for a *balanced* approach. They support using medications when necessary but emphasize lifestyle changes, therapy, and other holistic treatments as foundational for long-term healing. A short list of some of the most well-known voices in this space includes:

1. **Dr. Joanna Moncrieff** – UK psychiatrist, critic of the chemical imbalance theory, proponent of deprescribing and informed choice.

2. **Dr. Peter Breggin** – Psychiatrist known for warning about medication risks and advocating for non-drug-based treatments.

3. **Dr. Allen Frances** – Former DSM-IV task force chair; warns against overdiagnosis and casual use of medications.

4. **Dr. James Greenblatt** – Psychiatrist integrating functional medicine to reduce medication reliance.

5. **Dr. Ellen Vora** – Holistic psychiatrist prioritizing lifestyle and trauma healing over defaulting to meds.

6. **Dr. Mark Hyman** – Functional medicine MD, promotes root-cause approaches over lifelong medication.

7. **Dr. Daniel Amen** – Psychiatrist using brain imaging to personalize care and reduce unnecessary prescriptions.

8. **Dr. Drew Ramsey** – Integrative psychiatrist focused on food-based mental health strategies.

9. **Dr. Will Cole** – Functional medicine practitioner advocating for personalized, root-cause-based care.

10. **Dr. Robert Whitaker** (not a medical doctor, but a crucial voice) – Journalist and author of *Anatomy of an Epidemic* and other books, spotlighting psychiatric harm and supporting informed, patient-led decisions.

As Dr. Whitaker, an award-winning journalist, points out in *Anatomy of an Epidemic*, the rise of psychiatric medications correlates with an increase in legal disability rates. This begs the question: if prescription treatments are as effective as advertised, why are more people than ever struggling with mental health challenges and becoming increasingly disabled? The reality is that treating symptoms with medication alone can leave the underlying root causes unaddressed, perpetuating cycles of dependency, side effects, and even disability.

MOVING FORWARD MINDFULLY

We've spoken about the complex interplay of factors affecting a houseplant, analogous to human needs by way of our physiology, psychology, social connection, and spirituality. Our first step in making lifestyle upgrades is the best possible choice we can make, whenever possible. There may be some situations where you must 'medicate the plant' no matter what - sometimes people can't make the other changes first, and this is an informed choice that needs to be made alongside a highly qualified and board-certified professional.

LEARN THE SIDE EFFECTS AND COMPLICATIONS

If you're someone who finds sustained relief without significant drawbacks from medication, again, consider yourself blessed and lucky. For the rest of us, medications can feel like a revolving door of solutions that create new challenges. You are not alone in this struggle. I've been there, as have countless others. Medications can play a role in mental health treatment, but they are not the only tool—or even the most effective tool—for many people.

A balanced approach to mental health requires:

Informed Decision-Making: Before beginning a new medication, understand how it works, its side effects, potential for addiction or dependency, and its potential alternatives. Always research and ask questions.

Root-Cause Solutions: Along with pharmaceutical treatment, address lifestyle factors like sleep, nutrition, movement, and stress management. You'll hear more about lifestyle solutions in the upcoming chapters.

You are in charge of your body and mind, and with the right support, you can make informed choices that align with your values and goals. Being the CEO of your health care journey means only working with a medical professional team that empowers you, listens to you, validates your concerns, and believes you can thrive. Healing is not a one-size-fits-all process, but it is possible. Keep seeking, learning, and above all, trust your capacity to grow and thrive.

CHAPTER 3 SUMMARY

KEY CONCEPTS

1. **Stigmas in psychiatry.** Psychiatric visits are often designed to ensure patient anonymity, reflecting a cultural value of privacy and even secrecy. The more we discuss this topic with facts and normalization, the more we can progress.

2. **Acknowledge the quick diagnosis dilemma.** My own rushed diagnosis of bipolar disorder, based on limited context and without deeper investigation, led to immediate medication, a sense of lifelong mental illness, and a profound personal crisis. Diagnosing should be done over time, with care and precision.

3. **There's a bigger picture of pharmaceutical influence.** Parts of the healthcare system in many countries prioritize pharmaceutical profits over patient well-being. Psychiatry has been widely criticized for overmedicating and disregarding the root causes of mental health symptoms, something to be aware of.

4. **Taking a whole-person approach to medicine.** While corruption is rampant in the healthcare industry, a movement toward alternative, holistic care is growing. You can find medical professionals who value a whole-person approach to help you make informed decisions and find root-cause solutions.

QUESTIONS

1. When thinking of a whole-person approach to your health care, what areas of your lifestyle do you hope to improve or prioritize?

2. Think about the diagnoses you've been handed in your life. When you received the label, what were these diagnoses based on? Did you feel seen, heard, and understood in this process?

3. When, if ever, have you felt cared for by a health care provider? When, if ever, have you felt undervalued or dismissed? How did those experiences affect the way you view your health and what's possible for your future?

CHAPTER 4

BUILDING YOUR WELLNESS DREAM TEAM

"Who is wise? One who learns from all."

—Ethics of our Fathers

Several years back, in the heart of Jerusalem, two very different doctors offered me two very different versions of care. I was in the midst of a long, exhausting search—one that had spanned years and continents—for a doctor who could truly see me, listen with empathy, and help set me on the right course. I wasn't looking for a miracle. I was looking for someone who could help me connect the dots and support real, lasting healing.

One—an intuitive, functional medicine doctor—helped me reclaim my health in ways I never thought possible. But before I met him, I walked into a psychiatrist's office across town, hoping for a second opinion on my treatment plan. What I found instead was a jarring reminder of everything that's broken in the system.

The moment I stepped into his waiting room, I could hear every word he was saying to the patient before me. His sarcastic tone and sharp remarks instantly triggered alarm bells. My gut told me to leave. I didn't. (Note to self: never ignore that inner knowing.)

When it was finally my turn, this psychiatrist barely made eye contact. When I lowered my voice to speak, he laughed out loud and said, "No one out there can hear you," completely dismissing the reality I had just experienced. It was textbook gaslighting, and what followed was a cold, belittling exchange that left me feeling stuck, hopeless, and worse than when I arrived.

This was yet another episode in my saga with bad psychiatry. Immediately before this, I had met with a psychiatrist via Zoom during the pandemic—a doctor who prescribed me *seven* different medications without ever meeting me in person.

When I finally saw him in his office, it was clear to me that he was struggling with his own health—severe obesity, flushed skin, and a noticeable lack of energy were the obvious indicators. I don't share this to judge, but to underscore a realization that was becoming clearer with every interaction: I prefer to be guided by health practitioners who *embody* the vitality I'm seeking.

TEACHING BY EXAMPLE

While I fully respect that health can look somewhat different for each of us, I've come to deeply value learning from practitioners who walk the walk—those who live in alignment with the principles of whole-person health. The psychiatrist, who prescribed me seven medications virtually, showed no interest in exploring nutrition, movement, or stress relief as potential avenues for healing. Not once did he mention investigating root causes or looking at the bigger picture of my health. His approach was entirely pharmaceutical, relying solely on prescriptions as his tool of choice. When side effects emerged, he didn't reconsider the initial meds—he simply added more, creating what's been dubbed a "prescription cascade." No blood tests. No lifestyle recommendations. Just a quick diagnosis and a script to match.

Two years later, by chance, I ran into him at the gym. It looked like he was just beginning to incorporate movement into his life, being guided by a trainer. I found myself wondering—had he discovered the evidence showing that exercise can be just as powerful as an antidepressant for many people? Was he beginning to explore a new way forward? While I certainly wasn't planning to return to him as a doctor, in that moment, something clicked: the path I was seeking—one of vitality, integration, and root-cause healing—wasn't one he had yet walked at the time we met. And so, as well-intentioned as he may have been, he couldn't lead me to where he hadn't yet been.

Like many Western psychiatrists, his training was based in a narrow, pharmaceutical model—one that frames mental health almost exclusively in terms of brain chemistry and medications. But by then, I had already discovered a deeper truth: healing isn't just about suppressing symptoms. It's about restoring balance, from the inside out.

INDEPENDENT THINKING IN MEDICAL SPACES

When it comes to building your wellness dream team, it's important to remember how easily people, even well-trained professionals, can fall into patterns of blind obedience to authority. Consider, for example, this classic study:

In 1966, psychiatrist Charles K. conducted a groundbreaking study to examine obedience to authority in a hospital setting.[33] He wanted to determine whether nurses would follow a doctor's orders even if those orders could potentially harm a patient. As part of the experiment, a supposed doctor, "Dr. Smith," called 22 nurses and instructed them to administer 20 mg of a fictitious drug called "Astroten," despite the label clearly stating that the maximum daily dose was only 10 mg. Shockingly, 21 out of 22 nurses complied, violating hospital protocols and putting their patients at risk—all because an authoritative voice on the phone told them to.

While Hofling's study took place in the mid-20th century, one might assume that medical professionals today have become more independent thinkers, less likely to follow orders. Yet, recent studies confirm ongoing susceptibility for even highly trained professionals to obey orders blindly, even when those orders clearly cause harm. Psychologists like Megan Birney and her colleagues are also suggesting that something deeper than blind obedience is at play: what they call *engaged followership*.[34] In other words, people are more likely to comply with harmful instructions **when they believe they're serving a meaningful cause.**

This gives us a powerful insight: obedience often stems not from passivity but from identification with authority. This is why it is so important to stay conscious and discerning—not just of what we're being told, but also of *why* we're inclined to follow orders.

These obedience studies are so unsettling because they involve trained medical professionals with the knowledge and expertise to make better decisions. These nurses and healthcare workers had access to and knowledge of clear medical guidelines, but still deferred to authorities, ignoring their own judgment.

As consumers of medical care, this should give us pause—because **if seasoned professionals can override their own judgment in the face of authority, we must also be vigilant not to surrender our power or intuition at the expense of our well-being.**

CRITICAL INSIGHT IN THE PRESENCE OF AUTHORITY

Research on obedience highlights the deep-seated human hesitation to trust oneself in the presence of authority and the desire for approval from authority—even if that authority is acting recklessly or unethically. This pattern extends beyond healthcare and into broader societal issues, as history has repeatedly shown how masses of people, desperate for validation or fearful of dissent, will follow corrupt and dangerous leaders without question.

We need to be aware that even well-intentioned people are susceptible to the human tendency to obey without question. This is why it is important to maintain a Critical Insight when choosing and working with doctors, therapists, nutritionists, health coaches, and other helping professionals.

You can begin by asking yourself:

What are this person's motivations?

Do they benefit from my recovery? Or does their livelihood depend on my continued struggle?

Over the years, I've worked with dozens of practitioners—some of whom played a powerful role in my healing, while others, whether due to negligence or rigid thinking, became obstacles to thriving. The key difference between them wasn't their credentials—it was their *mindset.*

MINDSET

Mindset has become a buzzword across disciplines in the past two decades, largely due to the influential work of Dr. Carol Dweck, a Stanford professor, educational researcher, and author of *Mindset (2006).*[35] In her research, Dweck distinguishes between two fundamental perspectives: fixed and growth mindsets.

A fixed mindset assumes that intelligence, talent, and potential are static—you either have them, or you don't.

A growth mindset, on the other hand, recognizes that abilities can be developed through effort, learning, and persistence.

Our potential is *far* from predetermined at birth, something we'll further explore in chapter 6. Dweck's research confirms this: not only are intelligence and talent **not** fixed at birth, but the adoption of a **fixed mindset** *can* actually **reduce** potential—even in highly gifted individuals! Meanwhile, those who develop a **growth mindset**—embracing challenges, persisting through failure, and delaying gratification—consistently achieve the best outcomes in motivation, resilience, and performance.

Why, then, would anyone want to have a fixed mindset? A **fixed mindset** is often more convenient for the ego, seemingly allowing us to conserve energy. It allows people to say, *"I failed because I wasn't born talented"* or *"I can't do this because my IQ is too low"*—absolving them of the *effort* required to improve. There's also a subtle mindset trap, especially common among people who've been labeled as "smart": the fear that trying something new—and possibly failing—could shatter the image others have of them. So instead of risking failure, they avoid the challenge altogether. These ways of thinking provide easy escapes from the discomfort of effort and of failure, making the fixed mindset an alluring but dangerous trap.

YOUR MENTAL HEALTH PRACTITIONERS' MINDSET

When it comes to your **mental health**, adopting a **growth mindset** is essential. Acknowledging genetic predispositions and personal challenges is fine, but *we must never abandon the fundamental belief that growth* *and healing are possible.* It's far too easy to give up on ourselves when a figure in a white coat tells us that we're destined for a lifetime of illness. I know this all too well—I've fallen into that trap more than once, with devastating consequences. **Today I also know that the path to true healing begins when we refuse to accept those limitations and instead reclaim our ability to grow, adapt, and thrive.**

When choosing your healthcare and support professionals, it is essential to ensure that they have a **growth mindset**—one that recognizes your potential for change and improvement. Here are some questions you can ask yourself.

- Do they view your condition as a permanent, unchangeable reality?

- Do they believe in your ability to make meaningful lifestyle adjustments and enhance your mental well-being?

- Are they reinforcing a diagnosis as your fate?

- Or, are they empowering you with the belief that you can progress, heal, and thrive?

The mindset of your practitioner can directly influence your health outcomes—those who embrace growth will encourage you to take an active role in your recovery, fostering resilience and long-term well-being.

Just as individuals operate within a **fixed or growth mindset**, practitioners also fall into distinct **mindset paradigms**—and the one they adopt can have a profound impact on their health outcomes. At its core, this mindset determines whether a practitioner fundamentally believes in your ability to heal and grow or whether they see your condition as static and you as dependent on their services for the rest of your life.

Let's explore the two core practitioner mindsets:

1. **The Deficit-Oriented Practitioner**—This type of practitioner views you as fundamentally **lacking**—an empty vessel they need to **fix**. They place themselves on a pedestal, believing that **they alone** as the professional, hold the knowledge and solutions, while your role

as a patient is to comply and follow orders. They rarely consider your input, dismiss alternative perspectives, and prioritize authority over collaboration.

2. **The Asset-Oriented Practitioner**—In contrast, this practitioner sees you as a **whole, capable, and dynamic individual** with unique strengths and untapped potential. They do not define you by your diagnosis or challenges; instead, they recognize your **underlying needs** and offer their expertise as a **partnership** in your healing journey. They respect your perspective, believe in your ability to make meaningful changes, and encourage your active participation in the process. One key sign of an **asset-oriented** practitioner is their **openness to learning**—if you present a new avenue of healing, they will take the time to explore it rather than dismiss it outright.

The functional medical doctor who encouraged me to tap into purpose, is the perfect example of an **asset-oriented practitioner**. While his Harvard diploma hangs in his office, his focus is on his patients, not his credentials. On the other hand, the psychiatrist I saw across town was **deficit-oriented**. He had the shiny credentials, but belittled his patients and didn't listen to their concerns.

Choosing the right practitioner is about more than just credentials— it's about working with someone who believes in your ability to **function, heal, and thrive.** You're not entering a collaborative process if you go to the hospital to fix a broken arm. But when it comes to your mental health, so much about your health outcomes is in *your* hands, and it's of the utmost importance that your support team has an asset orientation.

When you're deciding on the right practitioners, stay mindful of how they make you feel in their presence. Here are some questions you can ask yourself.

- Do you feel respected? Empowered?

- Are they open to your ideas, and do they provide answers to your questions?

- Do they admit when they don't know something?

- Do they validate your feelings and thoughts with empathy?

- Are they solely focused on prescribing medications?

- Are they promoting your dependence on them, or your independence whenever possible?

- Are they teaching you (or at least pointing you in the direction of) skills and strategies to empower you to further your healing independently?

You've probably heard the popular saying that goes, "Give a man a fish, and you'll feed him for a day. Teach a man to fish, and you'll feed him for a lifetime." Interestingly, the Latin root of the English word "Doctor" is "*Docere*," meaning "to teach." One of the most empowering things a practitioner can do for you is to *teach* you over the course of your process. This includes pointing you toward a book, study, article, podcast, or any other type of learning that you can do independently.

A NOTE ON DEFAMATION LAWS

I've been frustrated over the years by the Prohibition of Defamation Law in my country, which prohibits people from saying or writing anything potentially degrading that could harm someone's livelihood. While I acknowledge there may be personality clashes between providers and clients, the negligence I've personally witnessed in certain instances over the years is inexcusable.

This huge gap in accountability can be attributed, at least in part, to the stringent defamation laws. People call me on a regular basis for recommendations to different care providers, so I know how many people are scrambling to find good help. I've wasted dozens of hours and too much money on this same search. **I look forward to the day when we will value patient health as much as we value professional livelihood,** and when we will have the freedom to share our objective experiences publicly to make the process of procuring a dream team that much more feasible.

FINDING THE RIGHT PRACTITIONER

Stay committed to your healing; you too will have the opportunity to work with asset-oriented practitioners who truly support your growth. I've been fortunate to work with several: the functional doctors who prioritize lifestyle adjustments, the psychiatrist who helped me taper off meds safely, and the functional health coach, Nomi, who set the tone in our very first meeting by letting me know that my story is what makes me interesting and not boring.

Nomi is not only highly educated—an encyclopedia of high-level science on human health—but she is also constantly learning, researching, and evolving. More importantly, she has an ASSET orientation: the ability to see potential in her clients and guide them to believe in themselves. **When you recognize the power that authority figures hold and the natural human tendency to defer to them, it becomes clear that anyone you trust with your well-being should have your best interests at heart.**

The asset-oriented practitioners on my journey have taught me how to trust my body, honor my intuition, and embrace healing as an active, collaborative process. *Remember, when choosing a practitioner, look for someone who sees your potential and respects your agency.* **Healing isn't something that's done to you—it's something that's done *with* you.**

Your story matters. Find practitioners who help you write the next chapter with clarity, compassion, and empowerment. The focus of your healing process is to guide you to your best possible levels of functioning. Practitioners hold a pivotal role in the healing journey, and the type of practitioner you choose can make or break your progress.

The **deficit-oriented practitioner** positions *themselves* as the hero of your story. They hold the knowledge, the prescription pad, and the so-called solutions, while you remain passive in the passenger seat—sometimes blindfolded.

In contrast, the **asset-oriented practitioner** makes *you* the hero of your own journey. And let's face it: you *are* the hero. *You* are putting in the effort, minute after minute, day after day. They share expertise, tools, insights, and strategies as you take the wheel. They believe in your ability to heal, and empower you to set and reach goals.

MEETING A TRUE HEALER

One of my personal favorite practitioners on the planet is renowned trauma psychologist and Holocaust survivor Dr. Edith Eger. She embodies the asset-orientation. I discovered Dr. Eger's work in 2019 on Oprah's podcast, when Oprah said she was "forever changed" by her book, *The Choice*.[36] After devouring Dr. Eger's books, taking her courses, and interviewing her twice, I will tell you that her wisdom profoundly changed my life.

Dr. Eger's story is beyond inspiring. She was only a teenager when she arrived at the infamous death camp, Auschwitz, with her mother and sister. Upon arriving, Dr. Mengele, the infamous 'Angel of Death,' asked her, "Is this your mother or sister?" When young Edie answered truthfully: "my mother," he sent her mother one way—to her death—and Edie and her sister in the other direction, to become prisoners in the barracks of Auschwitz.[37]

What followed was a nightmare of unimaginable trauma. Not only was Edie faced with the intruding thought that she had killed her mother with her response to Mengele on that fateful day, but time and again, Edie narrowly escaped death, struggling with starvation and abuse. Eventually, teenage Edie survived - barely living, rescued by American soldiers, from a pile of dead bodies, when the death camp was liberated on May 4, 1945. She would go on to face years of physiological and psychological trauma healing ahead. Her mother's words, whispered in the cattle car on their way to Auschwitz, would guide her path forward: "We don't know where we're going. We don't know what's going to happen, but always remember: **no one can take from you what you've put in your mind.**"

MOVING FROM SURVIVAL TO PURPOSE

Dr. Eger's healing took decades. She barely made it out alive from the death camps, and yet she went on to build a life of meaning and impact. She earned a Ph.D. in her 50s and became a world-renowned trauma therapist, helping people overcome their deepest struggles. She has worked with some of the most troubled people in society, including young people with hateful, neo-Nazi ideologies.

One of the messages that has empowered me the most is her teaching that "**anyone can live in a prison of the mind.**" Dr. Eger explains that for some, this prison of the mind can even be as miserable as her time in Auschwitz. When I first heard her say this, I was stunned. Growing up in a

Jewish family and learning about the Holocaust, and later marrying into a family of survivors, I'd acclimated myself to not "*kvetching*" (complaining) too much about my situation, because "it could always be worse," knowing that we have it good, compared to countless people who've experienced the horrors of the Holocaust and centuries of persecution.

While it's important to keep perspective on our challenges, hearing Dr. Eger describe how people can live in the "Holocaust of their mind" gave me something even more powerful: **permission to stop minimizing my own pain** and comparing my struggles to those that seemed more extreme.

Dr. Eger's teaching can free us from the psychological trap of comparison. **The truth is that suffering isn't relative.** Your pain is not diminished because someone else appears to have more. Your struggles can be addressed properly as soon as they're acknowledged as real and worthy of attention—no matter how insignificant they may seem in comparison to someone else's.

When I discovered Dr. Eger's teaching, I realized I had never fully processed the pain and trauma—not just of the symptoms I'd experienced since my teens, but of the treatment itself: the labeling, the hospitalizations, the sense of being defined and limited by a diagnosis. I had been minimizing my story for years, telling myself that all things considered, I was fine.

However, by listening to her advice and giving myself permission to see my circumstances as real, and also as hard—I was able to gain insight about my life, and ultimately process my past, coming out stronger for having done so.

It's okay to acknowledge that something is painful or difficult for you. It is okay to acknowledge that you are suffering, or even miserable, without comparing or belittling your situation by telling yourself that 'it could be worse,' or 'you should be grateful for what you have.' If you're identifying with this experience, you can ask yourself: what parts of your story could you acknowledge yourself for having lived through if you stop comparing yourself to other people?

TRUSTING YOUR INNER WISDOM

In my second interview with Dr. Eger, sitting next to her on a big white couch in her Southern California living room in the Summer of 2023, I asked her a question I'd been wrestling with, and in turn, learned a vital lesson about personal power. I couldn't wait to hear her reply when I asked her, "What do you tell people who have big dreams but are stuck in a perpetual cycle of self-doubt and impostor syndrome?"

At age 96, she immediately turned the tables on me in the sharpest fashion, making a lasting impression. "Let's do this," she answered, grinning warmly at me. "You be *me*, and I'll be *you*. What would *you* say to someone in this situation?" BAM. In that moment, she showed me that she believed in me and that the answers were already within me. **This is the essence of an asset-oriented practitioner—they guide you back to yourself, acknowledging your assets, and empowering you to trust your inner wisdom.**

BECOMING THE HERO

Waiting for external validation can feel safe, especially if you were raised in families and classrooms where adults judged and graded you. But true freedom comes when you learn to trust your own voice and make peace with your unique value. The only approval you truly need is your own. You too have tremendous inner resources, and by recognizing them, you can become the hero of your journey.

BUILDING YOUR DREAM TEAM OF ASSET-ORIENTED PRACTITIONERS

Here's how to identify and partner with practitioners who empower you.

1. **Do Your Research:** Look up their credentials, read their writing, and get a feel for their philosophy. Are they open to different types of treatments? Do they believe in your ability to thrive? If reviews are available online, read as many as possible and look for themes. Focus on what people are, by and large, saying about this professional, and their overall philosophies when it comes to mental health.

2. **Ask Questions:** During your first meeting, inquire about their approach. Are they open to non-pharmaceutical interventions? Do they view healing as a collaborative process? If medications, supplements, or protocols are suggested, ask about side effects, alternatives, and long-term implications of use. Remember, you are the CEO of your journey here, interviewing your prospective guides.

3. **Follow Inspiring Experts and Exemplary People:** Fill your eyes with inspiration. Whether reading books or engaging with social media or traditional media, surround yourself with practitioners and influences who uplift you. From fitness professionals to mental health practitioners, find voices that make you feel hopeful and motivate you to grow. The practitioner who also teaches is thereby empowering you to be independent, which is priceless.

4. **Focus on Solutions:** Surround yourself with people and resources that remind you of your potential. Rather than seeing your challenges as 'deficits,' reframe them as unmet needs. Stay vigilant that the right solutions are out there. You are the hero on this journey who will find answers and come out on top! Your healing journey is uniquely yours, but finding the right guides can make all the difference.

CHAPTER 4 SUMMARY

KEY CONCEPTS

1. **Be aware of the power of authority.** Despite their training, Hofling's obedience study revealed that medical professionals may comply with authoritative figures even when doing so violates ethical and safety protocols, underscoring the persistent need for critical thinking in healthcare. This is all the more so relevant when we are seeking care and in potentially vulnerable states.

2. **There's an impact of mindset on healing.** Dr. Carol Dweck's research on growth versus fixed mindsets demonstrates that belief in personal growth and adaptability is crucial for mental and physical well-being. It invites us to challenge the model that views conditions as static and unchangeable.

3. **Choose asset-oriented practitioners.** The key to effective healing lies in working with practitioners who empower you, respect your autonomy, and guide you toward self-trust and resilience, rather than fostering dependency and blind obedience.

QUESTIONS

1. Suffering isn't relative. Has minimizing your own suffering gotten in the way of your healing journey? How might acknowledging your past struggles empower you to heal and grow?

2. What attributes do you value in a medical professional or health care team?

3. Who inspires you to grow mentally, physically, and spiritually?

4. What are some non-negotiables for your dream team of health practitioners?

5. Think of someone you consider wise. What makes them wise?

OVERCOMING SHAME WITH THE POWER OF SELF-COMPASSION

"Shame dies when stories are told in safe places."

—Ann Voskamp

In the spring of 2013, I was drowning in shame, trying to recover from my first stay in a psychiatric ward. I had been thriving just months earlier—or so it had appeared. At 32, I had just begun a doctoral program while raising three young children, volunteering in my community, and running my practice as an Education Specialist. My schedule was relentless, and in my desperate attempt to keep up, I made a critical mistake—one with severe consequences.

Terrified that I wouldn't be able to manage it all, in the summer of 2012, I went to a general practitioner and asked if there was something that could help me stay focused and productive. After answering a few quick questions, I left with a prescription for stimulants. At first, they worked wonders. I felt sharp, energized, and capable. But soon, the same medication that was supposed to help me function began slowly but surely tearing me apart.

Within weeks of starting the prescription, I was using stimulants to jolt myself awake before dawn. Later, I'd take another dose just to push through my six-hour evening classes and the mountains of coursework each week. By 11 p.m. each night, I was still buzzing with energy. On the outside, my life looked golden—Dean's List grades, thriving clients, and a family life that seemed perfectly intact. I convinced myself I'd cracked the code for managing it all.

But beneath the illusion of success, I was juggling too many balls, including the fragile "glass balls" of sleep, self-care, and basic nourishment. And when those shattered, I shattered too—one sleepless night blurred into the next until I completely lost my grip on reality. I spiraled into full-blown psychosis and spent three weeks in three different psychiatric wards. I was away from my children for the entire duration, and the experience was by and large quite unpleasant.

When I emerged from the psych wards, I was heavily medicated, barely functioning, and drowning in shame. I took an extended leave from work and retreated from the world, convinced that if anyone found out what had happened, they would walk out of my life for good. I stopped answering calls and ignored texts, terrified that if anyone truly saw me in this state, they would lose trust in me for good. For so long, I had believed that my worth was tied to how well I performed, how much I gave to others, and how seamlessly I held it all together. Now that the façade had crumbled, I didn't know what remained of me beneath the roles I had played. I felt unworthy, unlovable, and irreparably broken.

And yet, one friend refused to let me disappear. She kept reaching out, again and again, until weeks later, I finally caved. Convinced she was inviting me out just to sever our friendship, I braced myself for rejection as I sat across from her outside The Coffee Bean on 3rd Street in Los Angeles, gripping my cup while elephant tears slid into my drink.

She studied me for a moment, then gently asked, "Is this what you've been doing all these weeks?"

Through my tears, I admitted that I had barely been able to get out of bed.

Then she said something I'll always remember: "Azi, you did not do anything wrong."

At first, I wanted to argue. I had done everything wrong—pushed my limits, skipped sleep, ignored my body, and convinced myself that asking for help was weakness. I had been juggling too much and pretending I could carry it all without consequence. I wanted to list every poor decision, and each moment I didn't stop, rest, or say no. I wanted to prove that I deserved the shame I was feeling.

But as her words entered my heart, something began to soften. **The truth was that I hadn't been reckless on purpose—I had been overwhelmed, ill-equipped, and doing the absolute best I could with the knowledge I had at the time. I wasn't a failure. I was a human being in survival mode, trying to hold everything together with a threadbare set of resources and an outsized sense of responsibility.** While this newfound realization didn't immediately erase my pain, something profoundly shifted in that moment. A small crack emerged in the armor I'd built, and compassion and empathy began to slip in through that crack.

For the first time in months, I felt a sense of relief.

Driving home, it hit me: forgiving myself wasn't just important—it was essential. If I truly wanted to heal and rebuild my life, I had to stop replaying my mistakes and start noticing the good I was still capable of—even in the smallest, quietest ways. I made a promise to myself right then and there: each day, I would write down three acts of kindness—whether for others or myself, including acts of self-care. It was a simple practice, but over time, it changed my relationship with myself, and in turn, with everything else.

By consciously acknowledging even the smallest positive actions, I began to rebuild my sense of self-worth and emotional freedom. As it's been said, "what you focus on, grows." I started by jotting down the acts on my Notes app each night before bed. In those early days, my "acts of kindness" were things like, "I got out of bed," "I gave my kids a hug," or "I walked around the block." But as the days passed, the list began to grow—and so did my strength. Learning to love myself again started with forgiving my missteps and affirming the seemingly small but meaningful steps forward.

THE TWO-WAY STREET

While mood, motivation, and mental states often stem from deeper physiological and environmental roots, the mind and body are in constant conversation. It's a two-way street. What we feed our minds, by way of both *what* we think and *how* we think, shapes everything: our physiology, our relationships, our daily choices, even our sense of purpose. Psychology is a vast and layered field, but in this chapter, we'll focus on a few of the most transformative mindset shifts—ones that have helped countless people, myself included, build a kinder, healthier, more empowered relationship with their inner world.

The mind doesn't operate in a vacuum—it's intricately connected to the body. Emotions are not just thoughts or feelings floating in space; they have biological roots. The nervous system, particularly the vagus nerve, serves as a communication superhighway between our brain and internal organs, constantly transmitting signals that shape how we feel, think, and respond. This means our mental and emotional states are profoundly influenced by what's happening in the body—from our heart rate to our gut health.

TRUTH: Just because symptoms are labeled as "mental" doesn't mean the imbalance *originates* in the mind.

Mental health challenges can be easily misunderstood, especially by people who haven't experienced them firsthand. For years, I struggled to articulate my feelings to people who simply couldn't relate. As I gained a deeper understanding of my own needs, over time I realized that effective communication starts with clarity—first with ourselves, and then with others. When you recognize that distressing symptoms and side effects aren't something you can simply "snap out of," it's easier to advocate for what you need, regardless of whether the people around you can relate.

If you've ever been asked why you can't "just snap out of it," know that the person asking likely doesn't grasp the depth of your struggle. I've had times in my life when, from the outside, I seemed to have everything—a loving family, fulfilling work, good health by many measures, and stability. Yet, I still found myself battling depression, anxiety, and even mania. I've learned that this incongruity of the external v. internal states isn't unusual. **Well-being—or the lack of it—isn't just a reflection of our external circumstances.** True mental health goes far deeper than what we have, what we've accomplished, or how we appear to others.

We live in an era of unprecedented material abundance and convenience, yet mental health struggles are more widespread than ever—even among those who appear to "have it all."

Take Robin Williams, for example—a comedic genius beloved by millions, known for his brilliance, warmth, and generosity. Despite the joy he brought to the world, he battled severe depression that ultimately led to his tragic death. Similarly, Anthony Bourdain—a charismatic chef and world traveler who seemed to embody adventure, success, and freedom—was silently struggling. His suicide in 2018 shocked fans across the globe, many of whom saw him as the epitome of a life well-lived.

These stories, among countless others, remind us that mental health is not determined by external success. True well-being is shaped by a complex interplay of psychological, physiological, social, and spiritual factors. And healing isn't a switch you can flip—it's a layered, nonlinear process.

While it may not qualify as a quick fix, understanding your own psychology can be one of the most empowering steps forward. When you learn how your mind works, what drives your patterns, and what your body might be signaling, you begin to access the kind of self-awareness that can support real, lasting change. In a world that is vying for your attention, paying attention to your inner world is one of the boldest steps you can take toward reclaiming your power.

WIDENING YOUR LENS

Gaining insight into your life story can profoundly transform your healing journey. For years, I saw my diagnoses of depression and bipolar disorder as life sentences—labels I had to hide, yet ones that continued to weigh me down, making everything in life feel harder. Over time, I realized that there is always another perspective. By reframing your perspective, even the most difficult moments can become valuable lessons that shape you into a stronger, more empathetic, and more interesting person.

How can we begin to reframe the most difficult parts of our stories?

Instead of viewing your symptoms or diagnosis as proof that something is "wrong" with you, try widening the lens. What else might also be true? What strength, wisdom, or insight has emerged from your experience? Whether or not you've realized it yet, the challenges you've faced have likely equipped you with resilience, emotional depth, and hard-earned tools for growth.

When it comes to healing, a single shift in perspective can create a ripple effect. While external validation can be uplifting, the most lasting change happens from within. Learning to love and accept your full story—not just the polished parts—is one of the most powerful healing tools you'll ever have.

I remember one of the emotionally toughest assignments from graduate school: writing a "failure résumé." We had to list our biggest personal and professional setbacks—a vulnerable and uncomfortable exercise. But the second part changed everything. Next to each failure, we had to write what we learned from it. That shift—seeing value in what once felt like shame—was transformational. It showed me that even our most painful chapters can become sources of clarity, compassion, and strength, if we're willing to reframe the narrative.

BEFRIENDING YOUR MIND

One of the most powerful psychological shifts you can make is becoming conscious of how you speak *to yourself* in your head and then guiding your inner voice to become more compassionate. This aligns with a concept called "Self-Compassion," which is the process of treating yourself with the same kindness and understanding that you'd offer to a friend facing the same situation. Dr. Kristen Neff, a pioneer in the field of self-compassion research, explains that there are three core elements in this process:[38]

1. Self-Kindness: Try to be more gentle and supportive to yourself rather than being harshly self-critical.

2. Common Humanity: Know that suffering and feeling inadequate are part of our shared human experience.

3. Mindfulness: Become aware of your emotions without judgment. Notice the thoughts and feelings coming up, and comfort yourself knowing that all thoughts and feelings are allowed without shame.

Research in the self-compassion approach shows that it can promote significant psychological benefits. People who practice self-compassion experience greater emotional resilience, reduced anxiety and depression, and greater satisfaction with life.[39] By speaking to yourself with the same empathy and support you'd offer to a friend, you can break free from destructive cycles of self-criticism and even self-sabotage, fostering a healthier relationship with yourself and bolstering your mental well-being.

LETTING GO OF SHAME

One of the most common and psychologically destructive emotions a human being can have is SHAME. Shame is the distressing feeling of unworthiness. While guilt is the feeling that you have *done* something wrong, shame goes much further, telling you that you *are* something wrong. Telling yourself, over and over, that there's something fundamentally wrong with you isn't just painful—it can be dangerous. A large-scale study of over 22,000 participants found that shame is even more strongly linked to depression than guilt, highlighting just how deeply this emotion can impact our mental health.[40] Shame takes a toll on mental health, and we definitely can't shame ourselves into healing. However, we can find our way out of the darkness and into the light with the power of compassion.

CHRONIC SHAME

Chronic shame, defined as thoughts and feelings of unworthiness over time, can hinder the ability to regulate emotions, lead to social withdrawal, diminish quality of life, and increase the likelihood of developing mental health disorders. However, no one is destined to feel shame indefinitely, and there are evidence-based strategies for breaking the shame cycle and learning to befriend your mind.

I know the destructive power of shame because I felt it personally for decades. My shame was classically disguised as the armor of perfectionism. On a deep and subconscious level, I blamed myself for foot injury as a toddler, and then for every single slight misstep of my life which happened after the injury, including my mental health rollercoaster. For the first decade of my adult life, I didn't disclose any of my mental health challenges to even my closest friends. That is how deep the shame around my diagnosis was. Over time, and with the strategies we're going to get into, I was able to let all of this go.

DEEPER LEVELS OF CONNECTION

Letting go of shame can be truly life-changing. **When we begin to recognize our shared humanity, it becomes easier to make peace with our own story, draw meaning from it, and even turn our pain into purpose.** The process often starts with small but powerful steps—like forgiving yourself and practicing self-compassion. It might also look like sharing your story with someone you trust, in a way that feels safe and right for you. When I first opened up to close friends about my mental health journey, I braced for judgment and rejection. But what I found instead was something unexpected: a deeper connection, greater understanding, and the kind of support I didn't know I needed.

What surprised me most after opening up was how many seemingly successful, happy people confided in me about their own hidden struggles with mental health. For years, I was convinced that sharing my story would push people away—but it did the opposite. Being honest about my journey didn't create distance; it created connection. Strangers began reaching out to say that my openness gave them hope—and in some cases, helped save their lives. This is the power of bringing darkness into the light: it doesn't just set *you* free, it lets others know they're not alone.

THE LONELINESS EPIDEMIC

Mental health diagnoses like Depression, Anxiety, Bipolar, and others are still widely misunderstood. Despite growing awareness, stigma continues to cast its shadow—fueling silence, shame, and compounding suffering. Right now, we are living through what many have dubbed "The Loneliness Epidemic," a time when its become the norm to spend more time on screens than in meaningful connection with fellow humans.

For those carrying the weight of a secret mental health diagnosis, that isolation can feel even more intense—amplifying shame and creating the illusion that no one could possibly understand. You know how heavy it can be if you've ever held a secret of this magnitude. So many topics become off-limits that genuine connection starts to feel out of reach. The secrets swirl around your mind in an inner dialogue, distracting you and disabling you from engaging with the person right in front of you. Loneliness, in these moments, isn't just about being alone.

Loneliness is the *feeling* of being unseen and unheard, and it happens even in crowded rooms on a regular basis. It happens when people keep significant parts of their stories to themselves. Connection and belonging happen when we can safely and securely share the parts of our stories that **matter most to our identity.**

MAKING PEACE WITH THE PAST

Making peace with the past becomes easier when we keep something vital in mind. As Greek philosopher Heraclitus so beautifully said, *"No man ever steps in the same river twice, for it is not the same river and he is not the same man."* Just as the river is always flowing and shifting, you are also constantly evolving—shaped by every experience and moment. Let the river metaphor settle in: you are not the same person you were yesterday. You are evolving—moment by moment, choice by choice—into something new.

Making peace with your mental health story starts with understanding what's really happening beneath the symptoms or diagnosis. As you now know, a label doesn't define you or reveal the full picture. Uncovering the root of your challenges may take time, but the key is approaching yourself with self-compassion and seeing your strengths, not just your struggles. Mistakes are part of being human; you can't rewrite the past, but you *can* free yourself from it. Acceptance, forgiveness, and taking the next step forward will lead you to emotional freedom.

ACTS OF KINDNESS JOURNALING

This is a powerful practice combining self-compassion and letting go of shame that you can implement to rewire your brain and see yourself in a new and more positive light. To start, take a few minutes at the end of each day to reflect on your positive actions—whether for yourself or others.

Write down three specific moments of kindness, self-care, or good choices you made that day. These don't have to be monumental; small actions like drinking enough water, taking a deep breath if you felt stressed, or offering someone a kind word all count. By documenting these moments, you begin to build "evidence" of the good you're doing and shift your focus away from self-criticism.

Over time, this daily practice supports neuroplasticity, strengthening neural pathways associated with self-compassion, self-efficacy, and positive self-perception. Each piece of evidence reinforces the identity of someone who is growing, caring, and making progress, no matter how small the steps may feel. With consistency, this practice can transform your inner dialogue and strengthen your sense of self-worth.

FILLING YOUR OWN CUP

By spring of 2013, I had completed an outpatient program at UCLA Hospital and was back in grad school, cautiously finding my footing again. As I reflected on what had led to my hospitalization, I began to recognize deeper patterns in my thinking. Pursuing a doctoral degree had always been my dream, but I hadn't fully acknowledged the toll that juggling so many responsibilities could take. Rather than stepping back from my other commitments, I sacrificed my own self-care just to keep up. Over time, **I came to understand that this wasn't only about ambition—it was rooted in a deep fear of disappointing others and, ultimately, losing them.** It took time to realize that caring for myself wasn't selfish but essential. As I've come to know, the truth is that we can only pour for others when our cup is filled. Prioritizing your health isn't a luxury—it's the foundation that everything else depends on.

A NEW APPROACH IN THERAPY

The next step in my healing journey was finding a good therapist to help me get through school smoothly and with as much mental well-being as possible. If you've ever looked for a therapist, you may know that this process can take time. Working with another person so intimately requires a level of trust, so you can feel safe and secure processing your difficult thoughts and feelings with someone who knows how to guide you to the other side. By this point, I knew that I needed an expert. After meeting two candidates, I nearly gave up. But on the third try, I found an absolute gem of a psychologist whose wisdom profoundly impacted my life. Dr. Patti Johnson's clinic listing online was called "Empowered Living." Her approach included an educational component; as a seasoned therapist and university professor, she felt strongly about empowering her clients with an educational piece so that they could understand tools and strategies for rewiring the mind and body.

Our work was mainly centered around a cognitive approach to therapy, which is focused on thoughts over circumstances. This approach was new to me. Previously, I had been under the impression that my childhood or my past was somehow shaping my present. Dr. Patti helped me to understand how, while we may on some level be dealing with repercussions of our past, *the most important piece in moving forward and growing is understanding and adjusting how we think.*

Cognitive-Behavioral Therapy, also known as CBT, is a goal-oriented and evidence-based approach to therapy. It focuses on helping the client gain awareness around and ultimately reframe thought patterns and behaviors to support positive change.[41] It rests on the idea that our thoughts, feelings, and actions are interconnected. In reframing unhelpful thoughts, we can thereby affect our emotions and behaviors as well. Some of the techniques used in this process can include journaling thoughts and evaluating those thoughts through a rational lens, rather than an emotional one.

TRAINING YOUR MIND

There is one exercise that I recall and still use to this day, any time I notice myself thinking in distorted, "all-or-nothing," "black and white," or extreme ways. An example of a distorted thought could be: "I'm a complete failure," or "things never work out for me." Dr. Patti taught me to use a percentage system to evaluate these distorted thoughts to straighten out my thinking and the moods that stem from those thoughts. Here's how I demonstrate this system.

THOUGHT-SHIFTING TECHNIQUES

This is the five-step thought-shifting process I've adapted from our sessions, and I find it can work wonders by way of shifting a mood.

STEP ONE: IDENTIFY THE THOUGHT

Write down a negative or distressing thought you're experiencing. For example, *"I'm going to fail my upcoming interview because nothing works out for me."*

STEP TWO: RANK THAT THOUGHT

On a scale of 0% to 100%, rate how much you believe this thought to be true. For example, you might initially rank it at 80% true.

Write down your evidence that the thought is true. In this case, it might be something like, "Well, I failed two job interviews in the past, so chances are this one will be the same."

Next, write down evidence to counter that thought. For our example, it might be something like, "I did get that job last year, and I had initially thought it would be out of reach. Plus, I've been preparing for this interview, which may prove helpful."

STEP THREE: REASSESS THE ORIGINAL THOUGHT
Based on the evidence in step two, reassess how true the thought feels now and assign it a new percentage. For instance, after reviewing the evidence, you might lower the belief to 40%.

STEP FOUR: REPLACE IT WITH A BALANCED THOUGHT
Write a more balanced thought that reflects the evidence. For example, *"While I might feel nervous for the interview, I've practiced and am prepared and have a decent shot of getting the job."*

STEP 5: GIVE THE THOUGHT A FINAL RANKING
Rate how much you believe the new, balanced thought on the 0% to 100% scale. This final step helps reinforce a healthier perspective.

MINDFULNESS THAT LEADS TO COMPASSION
The next step in healing my mind was learning about the world of Mindfulness. There are a few straightforward ideas and tools from this field that can help anyone get untangled from potentially detrimental thoughts. Mindfulness has become a popular word in recent decades, and in part, we can credit the flowering of Buddhist philosophy in the West. Similar traditions are found across several different ancient religions. The basic principles of mindfulness are universal, based in brain science, and can be practiced by anyone, including children.

Practicing mindfulness, the act of non-judgmental awareness in the present moment, literally changes your brain structure. Using advanced MRI scans, a 2011 study discovered that participants who completed an eight-week mindfulness program experienced measurable growth in brain regions that play a crucial role in memory, emotional regulation, self-awareness, and the ability to understand different perspectives.[42]

Mindfulness also decreases activity in the amygdala, the brain region governing your fear and stress response. By observing thoughts non-reactively, mindfulness practice has been shown to reduce activity in the brain's default mode network (DMN)—a region linked to rumination and self-referential thinking. This decrease in DMN activity supports improved emotional regulation and contributes to greater mood stability over time. [43]

The work of neuroscientist Dr. Richard Davidson further confirms that regular mindfulness practice fosters resilience and long-term well-being. His studies in experienced meditators also conclude that mindfulness increases the capacity to pay attention and sustain attention, as well as changing gene expressions related to inflammation and stress recovery.[44]

MINDFULNESS AND FEELINGS OF SAFETY

You can practice mindfulness on your own or with the assistance of an audio guide. For many people, and especially at first, silence can feel uncomfortable. It's completely natural to reach for background noise like the news, TV, or music to soften the mental chatter. It's a common way of coping, especially when our inner world is a whole new territory that we haven't yet explored. In mindfulness practice, the constant stream of inner thoughts is often called "the monkey mind." **The goal isn't to stop the chatter, but to observe it—to recognize that these thoughts are not *you*, and you don't have to believe or follow every one of them.** You are not your thoughts—and the more you learn to observe them without getting swept up in them, the more freedom you'll feel. At first, it might seem like your mood is tied to every passing thought, but with practice, you'll start to notice space between the two—and that space is where clarity and calm begin to grow.

You don't *need* to set aside formal meditation time to benefit from mindfulness. Simply paying attention to your thoughts—without judging them or getting caught up in them—is a powerful practice on its own. It might seem small, but this gentle awareness can create meaningful shifts in how you feel and respond to life.

I've led mindfulness sessions and seen how common it is for people to resist sitting in silence. I get it—before I started practicing, I resisted, too. And to be honest, I still go through seasons: sometimes, I enjoy the quiet, and other times, I find myself preferring background noise. It's all part of the process.

Before I ever tried sitting in silence with my thoughts, my mind felt like a whirlwind of self-criticism, judgment, fear, and shame. It's no wonder

I avoided it. One simple but powerful idea from evolutionary psychology helped me begin to break through that resistance.

SEEKING SAFETY IS HUMAN

As humans, we are constantly seeking safety—or at least the feeling of safety—because our autonomic nervous system is biologically designed to scan for threats and regulate our response to danger. This ongoing surveillance, known as **neuroception**, operates below conscious awareness and plays a key role in how we feel, behave, and connect with others.[45] **Seeking safety isn't a weakness—it's human.** Whether we're reaching for connection, structure, solitude, or control, so much of our behavior is driven by a biological need to feel safe. Becoming aware of this biological tendency can provide us with the opportunity to transform and evolve.

Safety seeking can look like creating daily routines, sticking to familiar environments, or practicing regular habits. Safety-seeking has a deeply social component as well, because building relationships and community provides us with both emotional and physical safety essential for survival. Safety-seeking can also look like excessively gathering information or over-preparing, for example, constantly checking the news, or exhaustively analyzing future scenarios to gain a sense of control.

When taken to an extreme, these types of safety-seeking behaviors can be time-wasting and even self-sabotaging, clearly not serving their intended purpose. A word of caution: the drive for safety can quietly morph into avoidance, perfectionism, or numbing—like socially isolating to dodge rejection, overachieving to avoid criticism, or escaping into food, substances, binge-watching, or doom-scrolling. These coping habits may offer short-term comfort, but they don't deliver the deep sense of safety your nervous system is actually craving. No matter how many safety-seeking behaviors you've engaged in, no amount of judging or shaming yourself will help you break out of these patterns.

The only way to upgrade your safety-seeking habits is by providing yourself with what it is that your human physiology is deeply seeking: *the feeling of safety.* So, if you sit down to practice mindfulness and notice your thoughts ruminating on your past actions, or you notice a craving to engage in a particular behavior, the best thing you can do is to soothe yourself and let your mind and body know that you are safe in this moment. This is an opportunity to practice self-compassion and speak to yourself as if speaking to a good friend in the same situation.

It can also be helpful to visualize a younger version of yourself, and speak to that child, letting it know that you will take care of it. As woo-woo as this may sound, the truth is that within every human being there is a child who, somewhere along the line, has felt unseen, unheard, and even unsafe. By accessing the wise and compassionate part of your adult self and speaking to the "inner-child" feeling unsafe, you can provide yourself with incredible emotional and psychological safety.

HOW TO PRACTICE MINDFULNESS

Lots of people find it helpful to follow along with guided mindfulness meditation tracks. Whether you're listening to audio tracks or practicing on your own, it can be helpful to start with a practice that focuses on two things: awareness and non-judgment.

Here's a basic overview of how to practice these skills on your own:

- Find a quiet enough place. Sit or lie in a comfortable position and gently close your eyes.

- Begin by softening your body. Gently release tension from the crown of your head down through your shoulders, arms, and torso, and all the way to the tips of your toes. Let your arms rest comfortably and feel their weight supported.

- Bring your awareness to your breath. Notice the gentle rise and fall of your chest and the sensation of air entering and exiting your nostrils.

- Choose an anchor for your attention. This could be your breath or—if your eyes are gently closed—a visual focal point such as the space between your eyebrows. When you rest your inner gaze there, you might start to notice gentle colors or geometric visuals beginning to emerge—like your mind is offering you something quiet, comforting, and just for you. You can focus on your breath or any other calming sensation, like the space around your heart.

- If your mind wanders—which it naturally will—gently acknowledge any thoughts without judgment, and bring your attention back to your chosen anchor. This isn't a sign of failure—it's part of the practice. Each time you return, you're strengthening your ability to focus and be present. You can think of thoughts as clouds drifting across the sky—observe them, then let them pass.

- Follow this practice for 5–10 minutes, or any amount time feels right for you. As it becomes more familiar, and if its helpful, you can gradually increase the length of your sessions.

NOTICING THOUGHTS

The ability to notice thoughts without engaging with them is incredibly powerful and becomes a skill you can use throughout your day whenever your mind starts drifting toward unproductive patterns. You can ask yourself, *"Is this thought important right now?"*—and if the answer is no, you can practice gently moving your attention to something else. While it's still a work in progress, this practice has helped me make peace with my thoughts, whereas before discovering mindfulness, my mind often felt like a courtroom, and sometimes even a prison. The mind has a tremendous capacity to transform our physiology, and by practicing mindfulness, you can literally re-wire your brain.

ONE MORE PRACTICE

There's another profound, science-based, and incredibly simple practice that can help you if you ever find yourself stuck in recurring, distressing thoughts, especially worries about upcoming decisions or events. In sessions with Dr. Patti, if I found myself perseverating over an event or future conversation, she would gently ask me, **"Could it be at all possible to wait until you get there, see how you feel, and then make your decision?"** This question can be revolutionary. So often, we plan and replay future events in our minds, imagining conversations or scenarios before they've even happened. But as the saying goes, *most of what we worry about never actually comes to pass.*

This approach can liberate you from the confines of your mind, reminding you that while planning and preparation have their place, obsessing over the future doesn't change reality. **Worrying about what's beyond your control is natural, but it's rarely worth sacrificing today's peace for tomorrow's uncertainty.**

By letting go of the need to pre-emptively solve every future problem, you may find more clarity, calm, and access to the present moment. What might be replaying again and again in your mind that you can let go of? What would happen if you let go of thinking about it now and wait to see how you feel when you get there?

While the practice of reflecting on this question is simple, to make it a habit, the best thing you can do is repeat using it, over and over. The habits that we practice repeatedly become easier and more automatic with that repetition.[46]

Your mind is not your enemy—it can become your lifelong companion with time and practice. Your mind can be shaped by experience and also reshaped by how you choose to engage with it. The stories you tell yourself about yourself have tremendous power. By replacing shame with self-compassion, fear with curiosity, and self-criticism with encouragement, you unlock a new way of living—one where healing is possible, growth is inevitable, and thriving is within reach. The journey is ongoing, but each moment of awareness, each small act of kindness toward yourself, is a step forward. You are not broken. You are becoming.

CHAPTER 5 SUMMARY

KEY CONCEPTS

1. **Mental health isn't just "in your head."** It's influenced by multiple factors and can be improved with self-awareness, thought awareness, and cognitive skills.

2. **Self-compassion is essential.** Speaking to yourself as kindly as you would a friend is a research-based practice that builds inner strength and resilience.

3. **Letting go of shame fosters connection.** Hiding struggles can intensify suffering, while vulnerability with discernment opens the door to deeper relationships.

4. **Prioritize mindfulness.** Practicing mindfulness can help you to see yourself as independent of your thoughts, rewire your brain structure, and provide you with the psychological safety that humans seek.

5. **CBT strategies can reframe thoughts.** Using a percentage system to assess the accuracy of distressing thoughts can help you adopt a more balanced perspective. You can also notice a worrisome thought and choose to delay thinking about it, shifting your attention instead.

QUESTIONS

1. How could reframing your self-talk affect your growth process?

2. Which habits, environments, or relationships help you feel safe and supported? And are the ways you protect yourself helping you thrive, or might some of them be keeping you stuck?

3. What supportive steps can you begin taking now to care for yourself with the same compassion you offer to others?

4. Are there parts of your story that you've chosen to keep private? If so, what might be influencing that choice—and how might it feel to share some of them with someone safe, when you're ready?

5. Letting go of shame begins with making peace with your past. If you could rewrite part of your story through the lens of self-compassion, what could change? What truth or strength might come forward?

6. Releasing the urge to solve every future potential problem can create more calm in the present. Is there a thought or worry that's been replaying in your mind? What could it feel like to gently let it go, even just for now?

PART 2
PHYSIOLOGY

CHAPTER 6

WIRED FOR WELL-BEING

"The body is the vehicle for the mind, and the state of one reflects in the other. Heal the body, and the mind will follow."

—Deepak Chopra, M.D.

For the first twenty years after receiving my mental health diagnoses, I believed what I had been told: that these "disorders" were lifelong and incurable. But over time, I began to question that narrative. And for me, healing the mind began—unexpectedly—with the body.

Flashing back to 2018, I was deep in postpartum fatigue, wrestling with depression, and dealing with a nagging ache in my foot that made even walking uncomfortable. I chalked it up to getting older, the aftermath of a difficult pregnancy, or maybe just the wear and tear of a long road with my mental health. I hadn't yet recognized the interconnected nature of the body and mind.

This shifted the day I first met my functional health coach and nutritionist. I'd been referred to Nomi, who worked in conjunction with my new functional MD. She listened closely, and I could feel that she really heard my story. Then she suggested something surprisingly simple: an anti-inflammatory nutrition protocol made up of nutrient-dense foods, a few targeted supplements, and some basic lifestyle upgrades.

I was skeptical, but Nomi struck me as practical, competent, and honest—and as someone who actually walked the walk. I wanted to believe her, and more than that, I was desperate to feel better.

Just three weeks later, so many things had changed.

The joint pain that had me holding on to the rails walking up and down my staircase was nearly gone. I could jog again—for the first time in several years. Even more surprising: I was waking up with motivation to be awake, and a sense of clarity I hadn't felt for a long time. In just 21 days, I experienced what I can only describe as a physiological awakening that was also influencing my state of mind. I was, day by day, witnessing the profound effect of physiological interventions to affect not only the body but also the mind.

THE MIND-BODY CONNECTION

When we talk about mental health, the focus often lands on thoughts, feelings, and behaviors. But as we've touched upon: your mental health doesn't exist in a vacuum. Beneath it all, your body and mind work together in deeply connected processes, shaping everything from your mood to energy levels to overall well-being. While constituting about 2% of your body weight, the brain uses an astounding 20% of the body's energy while in rest mode.[47] This means that around 1/5 of the nutrients and energy your body takes in will be devoted to brain functioning. While this puts the brain in a vulnerable place, what's exciting is that by making physiological upgrades in your life, you have a high likelihood of impacting your brain's functioning, which can lead to all sorts of improvements in your mental health and well-being.

By understanding the physiology of mental health, you can tap into a whole new world of healing and growth. The systems in your body, like sleep, nutrition, movement, hormones, and gut health, all influence your mental state. We need to work with these systems to heal and thrive. There are practical, approachable ways to make small shifts that can lead to big changes, helping you feel more energized, balanced, and in control.

THE HUMAN BODY

The human body is a miracle in motion. It works tirelessly—day and night—performing millions of complex processes so seamlessly that we often take it for granted. Beneath this incredible machine lies a profound truth: the state of our physical health is deeply intertwined with our mental well-being.

While the connection between the two isn't always at the forefront of conversations about mental health, science and personal stories show us that physiology can be one of the most direct and effective ways to improve our thinking, feeling, and functioning.

Consider someone like Tony Robbins. Long before becoming a global icon of personal development, he was struggling—overweight, depressed, and unhappy with his life, unsure how to turn things around. What changed? He started with his body[48]. By shifting his physiology—his nutrition, movement, and energy habits—he reignited his mind.

His transformation is just one of countless examples that reflect a deeper truth: **the body and mind are inseparable.** When we begin supporting our biology, everything else becomes more possible. I've experienced this in my own healing journey—how a few targeted shifts in my physiology opened the door to clarity, calm, and resilience I didn't know were available to me.

YOUR BODY: A SYMPHONY OF SYSTEMS

From the moment we exist, our bodies perform awe-inspiring biological feats—many of which science is still working to fully understand. It's biology, but it borders on magic. Without you needing to direct a single step, your body breathes, digests, heals, and balances thousands of functions in real time. At any given moment, **trillions of cells** are communicating and responding to your environment with astonishing precision.

Your immune system scans for invaders, your nervous system fine-tunes your responses, and your brain—just three pounds of tissue—processes more data than the most advanced computers on Earth. This internal symphony plays silently in the background, often without our awareness.

We may rarely pay attention, that is, until something goes wrong. A health scare, a diagnosis, or an unshakable symptom suddenly forces us to look inward. When it comes to mental health, the body's role is often underestimated—if not entirely overlooked. Yet if we want to truly thrive, we have to dig deeper. We need to understand how our biology, physiology, and daily choices shape the very foundation of our mental well-being.

THE HIDDEN POWER OF HABITS

Our modern lifestyles often work against the natural systems our bodies rely on. Evolution didn't prepare us for artificial light at midnight, diets full of processed foods, or endless hours seated at desks. Yet these very factors influence everything from how our cells function to how our minds process the world around us.

Building habits and simple daily practices that align with the body's natural rhythms can profoundly impact mental health. These include:

- Prioritizing sleep
- Eating more nutrient-dense foods
- Moving regularly
- Timed exposure to natural light

These aren't just wellness buzzwords; they're the foundation of how our systems were designed to function.

YOUR GENES ARE NOT YOUR DESTINY

For years, the prevailing belief was that genetics equals destiny. Your overall health destiny was viewed in light of your parents' genes, grandparents, etc. But groundbreaking research in a new field called "Epigenetics" shows how the environment and choices can influence gene expression.

Epigenetics is the study of changes in gene activity and expression that occur without altering the underlying DNA sequence.

These changes are influenced by environmental factors, lifestyle, and other external conditions, and they can affect how genes are turned "on" or "off." Through processes like methylation, certain genes can be turned on or off, giving us more control over our health than we once thought possible.

As we explored in relation to mindset, human potential is not fixed at birth. One of the most striking examples in biology is the well-known Agouti Mouse study.[49] In this experiment, researchers found that changing pregnant mice's diet altered how their offspring's genes were expressed. These changes impacted the pups' weight, coat color, and risk for chronic diseases—demonstrating that our environment can directly influence which genes get switched "on" or "off."

So what does this mean for humans? It means that your environment—including nutrition, stress, exposure to toxins, and even emotional experiences—can affect your gene expression. This can influence your risk level for mental health symptoms and conditions like obesity, diabetes, and cancer.[50] **Here's the hopeful part: gene expression can shift in the direction of resilience, vitality, and healing. You're not locked into the health patterns of your ancestors. With the right inputs, you can actively shape the direction of your own biology. Every nourishing choice you make—every breath, every moment of rest, every act of self-care—can lead to progress in your body. Transformation is not only possible, it's at your fingertips right here and now.**

THE RIPPLE EFFECT OF CHANGE

What's also quite fascinating about the Agouti mice study is that the epigenetic modifications observed in the mice could also influence subsequent generations, meaning that *maternal diet during pregnancy not only influences the baby in utero, but it also influences future generations that will be born to that baby mouse.* If this study teaches us anything, it's that the environment and influences experienced by one generation can have ripple effects well into the future. In other words, all the efforts you make on behalf of your own healing can have compounding positive effects, even in future generations. Genetics can offer valuable insight into your predispositions, but they do not define your destiny. While certain traits—like eye color—may be set in stone, many aspects of your health, including how your body responds to stress, inflammation, and factors related to mental well-being, can be influenced by your lifestyle and environment. **You have more power to shape your mental and physical health than you may have been led to believe.**

WHY PHYSIOLOGY MATTERS IN MENTAL HEALTH

Your body is a finely tuned machine, built to adapt, heal, and thrive. But when its systems are out of balance, the effects ripple through every aspect of your life—including your mental health. Addressing physiological factors isn't just about feeling physically better; it's about laying the groundwork for a healthier, more resilient mind.

From subcellular processes to the way our organ systems work together, our bodies hold the keys to unlocking greater mental and emotional well-being. The good news is that you don't need a degree in biology to make meaningful changes. Understanding and supporting your body's natural functions can create a foundation for lasting health and happiness.

Now let's dive deeper into how habits, environment, and physiology influence mental health—and explore practical, science-backed strategies to help you feel your best. The research is clear: the right mix of diet, supplements, sleep, exercise, and lifestyle interventions have the potential to slow biological aging.[51] [52] The connection between your physical habits and your mental health is profound—and incredibly empowering.

THE MIND-BODY LINK: BELIEF IS EVERYTHING

Here's the ultimate truth: your beliefs directly impact your physiology. What you *think* about your ability to heal and thrive influences your brain's wiring, stress hormones, and even immune function.

The placebo effect is a perfect example. When people *believe* they're receiving treatment, their bodies often respond as if they are—even if the treatment is inert. One of the most profound and credible studies on the power of the placebo effect was conducted at the University of Michigan. Researchers demonstrated that when subjects believed they were receiving pain medication, their brains released endogenous opioids—natural pain-relieving chemicals—and they experienced actual pain relief.[53] This study provides concrete evidence that the placebo effect has a *physiological* basis, not just a psychological one. It shows how powerful the mind is in shaping one's physical reality and, particularly, how beliefs influence the way one perceives experiences.

The powerful connection between belief and biology isn't limited to pain relief. Your expectations, perceptions, and mindset can influence a wide range of bodily systems—shaping everything from your mood to immune function.[54] Optimistic beliefs activate brain regions tied to motivation and reward, while pessimistic beliefs can increase stress hormones like cortisol, weakening the immune system. By thinking positively and believing in your potential to heal and grow, you lay the foundation for your body to follow along.

WHAT DO YOU BELIEVE ABOUT YOUR POTENTIAL?

What do you believe about your ability to grow, heal, and thrive? Belief isn't just a mindset—it's tied to a physiological process. Every time you reinforce a positive belief, you strengthen the neural pathways that make it your reality.

You can start right now by choosing thoughts that empower you—like "I can feel better," "I am capable," or "I can thrive." These aren't just affirmations—they're invitations for your physiology to hop on the transformation train. To help these thoughts stick, dig deep for real-life evidence that they're true. The more your body, mind, and soul perceive the *proof*, the more your belief becomes your baseline. This is how transformation begins—one powerful truth at a time.

If, for example, your new belief is "I am healing," look for evidence in your life that this is true, such as noticing improvements in your digestion, energy levels, cravings for water and healing foods, sleep improvements, and short moments of uplift in your mood.

Catch your body doing good rather than defaulting to noticing the negative. You can also mine for evidence in your past, reflecting on times when your body bounced back or healed over time, either mentally, physically, or both.

This is your journey, and you are in the driver's seat. Your body, mind, and spirit are ready to work together to create something extraordinary.

CHAPTER 6 SUMMARY

KEY CONCEPTS

1. **Remember the body-mind connection.** Physiological systems like sleep, nutrition, movement, hormones, and gut health deeply influence mental health.

2. **Consider habit realignment.** Modern environments can disrupt natural rhythms, contributing to stress and mental health challenges. Aligning habits with your body's natural

processes can profoundly impact mood and cognition. (More on how to do this is up next.)

3. **Your genes are not your destiny.** Epigenetic science proves that environmental factors can influence gene expression. This means you have more control over your health outcomes than previously believed.

4. **Belief influences biology.** What we believe matters. Optimistic thinking and self-empowering beliefs can rewire the brain, and in turn, the body.

5. **You are in control of your healing.** Even small, intentional changes in daily habits—such as movement, nutrition, stress management, and mindset shifts—can create lasting improvements.

QUESTIONS

1. What new truths could you begin to believe—truths that align with your highest vision for your life?

2. What signs—subtle or significant—can you recognize as evidence that you're healing, or beginning to turn a corner toward greater wholeness? What new truths might those signs invite you to believe about what's possible?

3. How might your daily choices—small, consistent steps toward well-being—create a ripple effect of healing, not just for you, but for future generations? What shifts when you see your habits as a legacy of health and empowerment?

FOOD AS MEDICINE: NOURISHING THE BODY

*"No disease that can be treated by diet
should be treated with any other means."*

—Rambam, 12th century C.E.

As a teenager in the 90s, I wholeheartedly bought into the lie of the low-fat craze. Having internalized the cultural value of thinness, my diet at 12 years old became a shrine to fat-free living: cereal with skim milk for breakfast, fat-free frozen yogurt at lunch, and pasta with iceberg lettuce salad and fat-free dressing for dinner. I remember feeling the pangs of constant hunger, never feeling truly satiated. My brain became a calorie-counting machine, so much so that I can still rattle off the nutritional stats of 90s snack foods without missing a beat.

Walking around deprived of essential proteins, fats, fibers, and nutrients is physically exhausting and mentally draining, and in my case, brought on feelings of anxiety and despair. Looking back, I wonder: if my after-school snack had been avocado toast with a few fresh organic eggs, instead of SnackWell's devil's food cookies, could I have avoided the crushing depression that crept in during those formative teen years? My best bet is that it may have helped. Reflecting on my own journey, listening to others who've experienced powerful mental health shifts through nutrition, and diving deep into the research, one truth keeps surfacing: **when we eat to support brain health, our mood and mental clarity improve—often dramatically.**

THE LOW-FAT LIE AND ITS CONSEQUENCES

If you survived the 90s, you may remember the "low-fat" craze of that era, too. Back then, cultural messages perpetuated the false notion that dietary fat was the villain, scapegoated as an unnecessary evil contributing to obesity and disease. Grocery aisles were filled with snacks boasting "fat-free" or "low-fat" on their labels. What *wasn't* advertised was that many of these packaged foods were *loaded* with sugar and chemicals —at levels that the human body could barely process.

The low-fat craze resulted from poor science and the corruption of individuals who put profit before people, which we'll get into shortly. So, there we all were in the 90s eating added sugar like it was organic kale and SnackWell cookies as if they were strawberries.

This low-fat era wreaked havoc on public health. Obesity rates doubled between 1980 and 2000, and heart disease soared.[55] Less obvious, but equally devastating, were the mental health consequences. By the mid-2010s, research revealed a stark connection: inadequate healthy dietary fat—critical for brain health—was linked to depression.[56] By 2012, findings from the food and mood data of over 9,000 men and 3,000 women between the ages of 45 and 60 concluded that higher adherence to low-fat, Western, high-snack, and high fat-sweet diets was associated with an increased likelihood of depressive symptoms, while traditional and healthy dietary patterns were linked to a lower likelihood of such symptoms.[57]

THE SUGAR EPIDEMIC

If you were to walk into any store selling tobacco products in a number of countries today, you'd find walls of cigarette boxes plastered with bold black labels and bright red warnings.[58] You won't see any colorful camels or cool cowboys on the labels. There is not one beautifully branded package in sight on these tobacco shelves, because of laws mandating standardized packaging with clear warning labels that smoking is dangerous and even deadly.

Flash back to the mid-20th century, cigarette companies used to advertise smoking as a healthy habit, with some brands even featuring endorsements from medical doctors. A 1946 R. J. Reynolds Tobacco Company advertisement claimed, "More doctors smoke Camels than any other cigarette."[59] Nearly eighty years later, we are experiencing another health epidemic caused by a dangerous substance, which, while this may be hard to swallow, has also been falsely endorsed as healthy.

This newer health epidemic has striking similarities to the tobacco scandals of the 40s. Just twenty years after doctors were publicly endorsing smoking, two Harvard scientists by the name of Dr. Fredrick Stare and Dr. D. Mark Hegsted were paid $6,500 (the equivalent of $50,000 in 2024) by The Sugar Research Foundation (today called the Sugar Association) to downplay the role of sugar in causing heart disease, instead pointing a finger to dietary fat as the main culprit.[60]

The Harvard scientists published their falsified findings in The New England Journal of Medicine in 1967, without disclosing the sugar industry's blatant sponsorship. This strategic move influenced public perception and dietary guidelines, diverting attention from sugar's health risks for decades.

To make the sugar story even more complex, we now know that major tobacco companies—like Philip Morris and R.J. Reynolds—expanded into the food industry in the late 1980s, creating many of the highly processed, sugar-laden foods that dominate store shelves today.[61]

These corporate acquisitions and the marketing strategies that followed are infamous for transferring marketing tactics originally used to target ethnic and racial minorities directly into the processed food and beverage industries. These tactics were intentionally aimed at vulnerable populations. The extent of public deception behind the production and marketing of processed foods is hard to stomach.

To be clear, swapping healthy dietary fat for processed sugar is not like swapping apples for oranges; it expedites a propensity for harmful sugar addictions, and here's why. Dietary fat is what helps you feel satiated, stabilizes blood sugar, and reduces cravings for more food.[62] When people stopped eating dietary fat, a sugar epidemic began in full swing.[63]

WHAT DOES SUGAR DO TO THE BODY?

What exactly is the issue with sugar when it comes to mental health? High levels of sugar consumption are correlated with depression, evidenced by a 2024 study which found that each additional 100 grams of daily sugar consumption increases the prevalence of depression by 28%.[64] Consuming refined carbohydrates and added sugars can also cause *reactive hypoglycemia,* a phenomenon caused by rapid increases in blood glucose, followed by significant drops. This sugar crash can cause intense carbohydrate cravings, fatigue, brain fog, and even anxiety.[65]

Sugar is not just sparkling white crystals in cute little rectangular packages. It is hidden in plain sight, even inside foods labeled as healthy.[66] Currently, 74% of all items in US grocery stores contain added sugar.[67] For the consumer, this isn't always easy to notice. UCSF scientists explain in their report on sugar, *Hidden in Plain Sight:* "There are at least 61 different names for sugar listed on food labels. These include common names, such as sucrose and high-fructose corn syrup, barley malt, dextrose, maltose, and rice syrup, among others."[68]

The World Health Organization (WHO) recommends limiting our daily intake to 25 grams of added sugar for adults.[69] While this may sound like a decent amount, eating just one package of some yogurts or one glass of juice can put you over the limit.

REDUCING SUGAR INTAKE

If there is ONE thing you can upgrade in your nutrition plan to alleviate symptoms of depression right now, it's replacing sugars with more nutritious foods. A 2015 study examined the effects of added sugar simply by removing it from the diet of 43 children with obesity and metabolic syndrome.[70] Their calorie intake was maintained - this was not a weight-loss diet, and the children were not being fed the healthiest foods on the market, or even extra vegetables. It was a nutritional study taking out just one variable from their diets, and what happened over the course of nine days was striking.

Parents observed that their children were irritable and difficult for the first five days, likely due to withdrawal from sugar and fructose. However, after the initial adjustment phase, parents, teachers, and the children themselves noted positive changes. The children demonstrated improved concentration, better school performance, reduced irritability, and overall behavioral improvements. Many children described feeling mentally clearer, stating it was the first time they felt their minds were not "clouded."

These findings are crystal clear: reducing sugar intake can lead to significant cognitive and emotional benefits. The children showed significant improvements in their overall health in metabolic health markers, including reductions in blood pressure, fasting blood glucose, insulin levels, and liver fat.

If this science is so clear and we know that added sugar is creating behavioral, mental health, and overall health complications, why, then are 92% of US school food programs exceeding the recommended limit for added sugars at breakfast, and 69% at lunch?[71] The leading culprit in exceeding the sugar limit turns out to be flavored milks, hiding sugar beneath a guise of health. Something is *extremely* awry here.

The WHO estimates that 5% of all the people on the planet are clinically depressed[72], while in America, this number is multiplied, ranging between 10 and 27%, based on location.[73] America also happens to be the largest per capita consumer of added sugar, now coming in at 126 grams per day per person, several times the recommended limit.[74] This statistic is especially alarming given that the recommended maximum intake is just a fraction of that amount. When you consider the profound toll this excess is taking on the mental health of an entire society, it begs the question: **Can the short-lived pleasure of sugar possibly be worth the cost in quality of life?**

THE SUGAR AND MENTAL HEALTH CONNECTION

When it comes to sugar and mental health, we need to understand what's happening beneath the surface. Robert Lustig, Professor of Pediatric Endocrinology and expert in public health, provides a clear explanation for the brain science of sugar addiction.[75] He explains that *pleasure* and *happiness are commonly confused*. The difference between these two pursuits affects our neurochemistry and mental health. The line between pleasure and happiness can become blurred in the mind, but understanding the difference is essential in the process of reclaiming your mental health.

PLEASURE AND DOPAMINE

Much of modern life is wired to keep us chasing dopamine, one quick hit at a time—from ultra-processed foods to social media scrolling and the constant pinging of digital devices. At the heart of this chase is dopamine, a neurotransmitter responsible for reward, motivation, and the drive to act. Dopamine isn't the enemy—it's your brain's way of keeping you driven and on task.

The trouble with dopamine starts when we overstimulate it. Over time, our brains can build up a kind of tolerance, meaning we need more and more stimulation just to feel the same spark of satisfaction.[76] Constant hits—like endless scrolling, snacking, or juggling a dozen tabs at once—can wear down our natural reward systems, making it harder to feel calm, focused, or even content.

When the brain's reward system gets bombarded too often, it starts to dial things down. Dopamine receptors become less sensitive, which means everyday pleasures don't hit like they used to. This can leave us chasing stronger and stronger stimulation just to feel okay—and that's how we end up in burnout or stuck in patterns that look a lot like addiction.

HAPPINESS AND SEROTONIN

Happiness, on the other hand, is connected to a different neurotransmitter, called serotonin. Serotonin plays an important role in regulating mood, and in the right amounts, promotes contentment, connection, and sustainable feelings of well-being. It's also much less likely to lead to addictive behaviors. Serotonin is fostered by cultivating meaningful relationships, volunteering, and practicing gratitude.[77]

Interestingly, about 90% of your body's serotonin is made in the gut—mainly by the cells that line your digestive tract.[78] Since serotonin is made from the essential amino acid tryptophan, which we can only get through food, feeding our bodies with the right nutrients plays a key role in supporting healthy brain function. Here's the twist: constantly chasing dopamine highs can actually disrupt serotonin balance—making it harder to feel calm, content, or genuinely happy. This is why addiction can feel so miserable, especially over the long term.

Sugar has a pronounced effect on dopamine receptors, and while it may produce pleasure in the short term, the chemistry behind the scenes is potentially making happiness and thriving more and more out of reach as consumption increases.[79]

I'm not here to tell you to cut sugar out completely—what you choose to eat is entirely up to you. But here's the thing: when it comes to sugar, the real power lies in being informed. Once you understand what it's doing to your body and mind, you get to make decisions from a place of awareness—not habit or misinformation. And that's where freedom begins.

Just like cigarettes are packaged with health risk dangers, written loud and clear on the packaging in many countries, you can imagine what kind of extreme health warnings would be on most packaged foods if only "Big Food" (the food industry) had your best interest and well-being in mind more than their profiting from selling addicting substances. If this were the case, you'd be seeing labels such as this one: *High consumption of ultra-processed foods has been linked not only to increased risk of all-cause mortality, but also to a wide range of chronic health conditions—including depression, anxiety, cognitive decline, metabolic syndrome, obesity, and cardiovascular disease.*

Whether you're ready to lower your consumption or ditch the added sugars in your foods entirely, you'll appreciate that *adding* nutrients can also improve mood and well-being. In a double-blind study of 231 prisoners, Cambridge University researchers studied the aggressive behaviors of prisoners before and after essential nutrient supplementation.[80] After taking capsules of vitamins, nutrients, and essential fatty acids for two weeks, violent behavior decreased by 35%. The prison supervising medical team reported no adverse effects whatsoever from the supplements. Nutrients influence not only our bodies, but also our minds. You can literally look at food not only as fuel but also as medicine. The connection between food and mental health isn't just theoretical—it's personal.

OUR SHARED HISTORY OF FOOD AS MEDICINE

For centuries and across cultures, food has been used as a primary form of medicine. Ancient texts detail how certain plants heal ailments, from physical pain to emotional distress. Nutritional wisdom was passed down through generations, shaping how we cared for our bodies and minds. But in the early 20th century, so many things changed. On one hand, the development of safer pharmaceutical cures revolutionized healthcare.

At the same time, as medicine modernized, our reliance on food and nature waned. The industrial age brought quick fixes: Tylenol for headaches, Valium marketed to stressed-out moms in the 1960s, and later, opioids marketed as essential for pain management. While Western medicine has achieved extraordinary breakthroughs in many arenas, it has also led us to prioritize instant relief over long-term, sustainable solutions. The results we're seeing, by and large, are societies often treating symptoms instead of addressing root causes, relying on pills and processed foods instead of lifestyle changes and natural remedies.

HOW NATURE WAS SIDELINED BY INDUSTRY

It's important to keep in mind how we got here. Back in the early 1900s, something big happened that I certainly didn't learn about in school. A report called the **Flexner Report**, funded in part by the **Rockefeller Foundation**, changed the entire direction of medicine in the West. With a focus on "modernizing" medicine, traditional healing methods—like plant medicine, nutrition, and holistic care—were labeled as unscientific or even dangerous "quackery."[81]

The system was restructured to favor pharmaceutical drugs and profit-driven care. Natural and time-tested healing approaches were pushed to the sidelines, while chemical-based treatments became the gold standard. Simply put, Rockefeller's influence helped turn medicine into big business.

The impact? Generations have grow being told that only pills can fix what's wrong—and that anything outside the mainstream must be nonsense. But now, with immediate access to transparent information, we can wake up to the beautiful truth: reconnecting with the benefits of nature can play a powerful role in our health and well-being.

WHAT WE KNOW NOW

We now understand that mental health isn't just "in your head." It's deeply connected to your body, including what you eat. Nutritional psychiatry is uncovering powerful links between diet and mood, showing how certain foods can even fuel resilience, while others exacerbate depression and anxiety. The takeaway is simple yet profound: food is more than calories. It's information for your cells, fuel for your brain, and the foundation of your overall well-being. Had I known then what I know now, and had someone asked about my diet instead of handing me a prescription, my story would have taken a very different turn.

FROM DIETING TO THRIVING

Since my depression diagnosis in 1995, I've tried nearly every diet under the sun: low-fat, high-protein, low-carb, raw food, vegan, ketogenic, you name it. In my younger years, it was for the potential physical outcomes, namely losing a few pounds. As a teen with a medium build in a society that valued extreme thinness, the pressure to be thin was intense. Because of my chronic foot pain issue, I wasn't able to exercise comfortably and get my heart rate up often enough, leading to a lack of exercise. I am certain that this contributed to my depression symptoms.

For years, I thought dieting was about willpower. But I've come to understand that true health, and sustainable weight, is a side effect of properly fueling and working with both the brain and body. The problem isn't your discipline; it's the diet industry's empty promises. Yo-yo dieting doesn't just fail you emotionally. It slows your metabolism and makes long-term health harder to reach.

If you've ever tried a diet and failed, you are certainly not alone. A 2022 study from The Ohio State University Wexner Medical Center found that approximately 95% of dieters regain the weight they lost within two years.[82] With that being said, if you've resigned yourself to the assumption that you'll always crave sugar or that you need to restrict yourself and experience some level of suffering around food, I want you to know that there are alternatives. Until I learned to eat for my brain health, I mistakenly believed that craving processed sugars was an inevitable part of human existence. Over time, I've internalized the fact that this simply isn't true.

NUTRITION: YOU REALLY ARE WHAT YOU EAT

When you eat, you're not just fueling your body. You're literally rebuilding it. Each bite is broken down into molecules that your body uses to create cells, tissues, and energy. **Take a handful of almonds, for instance:** as you chew, you break down the cell walls, releasing proteins, healthy fats, and micronutrients. These nutrients travel through your digestive system, are absorbed into your bloodstream, and eventually nourish your cells. They are literally becoming part of your body. Your body is constantly rebuilding itself, and the quality of the "building blocks" you provide, like nutrient-dense foods, directly impacts your energy, mood, and overall well-being.

YOUR JOURNEY WITH FOOD

The key to using food as medicine is to educate yourself, get curious, heal, observe (ECHO), and find what works for *you*. While certain principles, like prioritizing whole, nutrient-dense foods, benefit most people, your optimal nutrition plan will depend on your unique needs, preferences, and goals. The key here is finding your harmony by leveraging the incredible advancements of modern medicine, while honoring the ancient and proven wisdom of food as a tool for healing.

Now that you understand the importance of nutrition, let's take stock of your daily eats. You can rest assured that the process of upgrading does not need to be painful or feel restrictive. When done right, it can leave you feeling incredibly satisfied and energized.

Remember, the goal here is to guide you into thriving and feeling your best. I'm intimate with the pain of diet deprivation, and plans focused solely on eliminating things. So, the approach we're going to take is to focus on what you're adding to your brain and body through the foods you'll consume.

MAKING MEANINGFUL CHANGE

Changing how we eat isn't always easy. What I've learned, both through research and firsthand, is that the hardest part isn't swapping food. t's the feeling of fear. If we anticipate feeling deprived, restricted, or hungry, there's a fear that can hold us back before we even begin. By now, you may be realizing that this experience of feeling plays into the power of *belief*. What we believe about food, and what we expect to feel, can shape our experience. Rest assured, a plan for sustainable thriving will help you feel better and ditch the craving-hunger roller coasters that happen so often with regular high sugar or ultra-processed food consumption.

What you need to remember here, and with any upgrade you're making, is that you may fall in love with the upgrade and all your new healthy foods straight out of the gate. Or it may be that finding foods you love takes multiple exposures, experimenting with a few recipes, and giving your body time to acclimate by eating differently. For most people, lasting change takes time. Give yourself grace with this process.

Here are some practical tips to recalibrate your body and set yourself up to feel great and thrive:

- Start by adding lemon or apple-cider vinegar water to your mornings and hydrating throughout the day.

- Start your day with savory foods. Include veggies, protein, and healthy fat. This will help you avoid a morning glucose spike, leading to cravings and fatigue later in the day.

- Avoid eating sugary or carbohydrate-rich foods on an empty stomach.

- Begin each meal by eating high fiber veggies to slow glucose absorption.

- Instead of denying yourself something you're craving, first give your body the nutrients it needs and wait to see how you feel. This may help you feel less interested in the less nutrient-dense foods later.

By doing all of these things, you're slowing the body's glucose absorption, stabilizing energy, and reducing the chance of later cravings.

MEAL PREPPING TO PRIORITIZE NUTRITION

Let's face it. Even on a good day, prepping three healthy meals can feel like a task. For many folks, the convenience of processed foods often wins out, but at a cost. While I'm all for convenience, I'm also a realist, acknowledging that the time spent prepping food can have big payoffs for energy, health, and mood in the long run.

Instead of feeling sluggish or sick hours (or years) later, the time investment in prepping food will pay you back with both time and energy. You don't need complicated recipes, and you can keep your processes simple.

I want to level with you if you're accustomed to packaged or fast foods. Home-cooked meals or healthier menu options might not look appealing to you at the beginning of your process. Over time, as hard as it may be to believe, you can come to crave and even prefer them. The good news for everyone is that it doesn't take long for the body to adapt. Your body knows what it needs, and your job is to give it a chance to realign.

It's true that the quick hit of pleasure from a sugary snack or fast food can feel good in the moment. But over time, the deeper satisfaction comes from making choices that truly nourish you. We all may feel a tendency to trade long-term well-being for short-term gratification, but the more we recognize that pattern, the more power we have to choose differently. By honing your non-judgmental awareness, you can kindly guide yourself to make more wellness-affirming choices.

CHAPTER 7 SUMMARY

KEY CONCEPTS

1. **The sugar industry has influenced public opinion.** In the 1960s, it manipulated scientific research, misleading the public, shaping decades of flawed nutritional guidelines, and causing a sharp decline in health outcomes.

2. **Sugar deeply affects our mental health.** Excessive sugar intake is linked to increased risk of mood disorders and cognitive issues. Eliminating processed sugar can rapidly improve behavior, focus, and emotional well-being.

3. **You are what you eat.** You're not just fueling your body with nutrient-rich foods. You're rebuilding it, one choice at a time. Focus on what you're adding in, and trust that small, intentional steps like lemon water in the morning, a protein-rich breakfast, or weekly meal prep, can make a lasting impact on your energy, mood, and well-being.

QUESTIONS

1. Does understanding the link between nutrition, mood disorders, and cognitive issues shift your thinking about what you want to eat?

2. Take a moment to reflect: what messages did you receive about food as a child? How have those beliefs evolved over time?

3. What could be a new area of growth for you when it comes to nourishing your body? Write down your thoughts, acknowledging them is a powerful first step toward creating lasting, positive change in your relationship with food.

4. What excites or inspires you to nourish your body in ways that support your mental and physical well-being? What gives you hope or motivation to make lasting shifts? Jot down your thoughts, and you can return to them whenever you need a reminder of why this is so important.

CHAPTER 8

GUT HEALTH: YOUR INNER-DINNER PARTY

"The gut is not like Las Vegas. What happens in the gut does not stay in the gut."

—Alessio Fasano, M.D.

In 1995, at 15 years old and with a belly full of fat-free food, I was officially diagnosed with clinical depression. Like a majority of mental health disorder diagnoses, mine was made in an approximately 15-20 minute visit with a general practitioner.[83] Back then, depression wasn't a topic of mainstream conversation. The ride to the doctor's office with my mom was silent; the air was thick with my unspoken shame.

In the waiting room before my appointment, I filled out the 21-question Beck Depression Inventory (BDI). The BDI is a widely used self-report questionnaire that has been in use since the 1960s to diagnose depression and assess its level of severity.[84] It assigns a numerical value to specific symptoms, such as mood, levels of pessimism, sense of failure, self-dissatisfaction, guilt, and suicidal thoughts. Notably, it doesn't account for any potential physiological root causes of these symptoms.

The BDI (Beck Depression Inventory) asks you to rate your experience on a scale of 0 to 3, with 3 reflecting the most severe symptoms. I remember carefully filling in mostly 2s and 3s—being honest, at first. But then I paused. I erased some of the 3s and changed them to 1s. I didn't want to alarm my parents or make anyone worry about me. I was already overwhelmed, and the thought of adding guilt to the mix felt unbearable.

After tallying my score, the doctor looked up and said, "You're moderately depressed," then handed me a prescription for Prozac. Had I answered honestly, my score would've landed in the severe range. But even then, there was no conversation about what might be driving my pain. No questions about my nutrition, lifestyle, sleep, movement, trauma, or support system. Just a label, a pill, and a quick, "Feel better—follow up in three months."

THE GUT-BRAIN CONNECTION

What we didn't know during the low-fat 90s craze was how much this trend disrupted gut health, and thereby brain health, and mood. By filling up on processed, fat-free "foods," the gut microbiome—the ecosystem responsible for producing 90% of the body's serotonin—is thrown completely out of balance.

Today, we understand the critical role of the gut in serotonin production.[85] [86] As we've touched upon, most of our serotonin is made in the gut's enteric nervous system (ENS), often called our "second brain." Enterochromaffin cells in the gut manufacture serotonin, which not only influences digestion but also plays a key role in mood and mental health via the gut-brain axis. Like an information highway, the vagus nerve connects the gut and brain, sending signals that shape how we feel emotionally and physically.

The bottom line is that an imbalanced gut can lead to serious repercussions for mental health. Enter *psychobiotics*, an emerging field exploring how gut bacteria influence mood and mental well-being, offering new hope for those struggling with mental health challenges.

Psychobiotics looks at how beneficial bacteria (probiotics) and fiber-rich foods (prebiotics) support gut health and, in turn, improve mood and mental well-being by influencing the gut-brain connection.[87] Research shows that eating fermented foods—like yogurt, kimchi, and sauerkraut—alongside fiber-rich options such as beans and leafy greens, can boost the production of neurotransmitters like serotonin, which support happiness and relaxation. Think of it as a two-for-one deal: improving your gut health *and* strengthening emotional resilience.

HOW IT WORKS

As we've explored, the brain and gut are linked through a powerful, two-way communication system. What may surprise you is that most of the messages actually travel from the gut to the brain—not the other way around. Far beyond digestion, the gut is a central player in immune function and mental health, acting as a communication powerhouse via the vagus nerve.[88]

Think of your gut as hosting a dinner party with diverse bacteria, each with its own preferences. Some love sugar (those are the "small-talk type" guests), while others thrive on fiber and nutrient-rich foods (your "deep conversation type" guests). If you only feed the sugar lovers, the meaningful guests might stop showing up, and your party—aka your gut microbiome—loses its balance. A diverse, well-fed microbiome supports better mental health, reduces cravings, and promotes resilience.

DEPRESSION AND GUT HEALTH

At the time of my diagnosis of depression, it was widely considered a "chemical imbalance" of serotonin in the brain, based on the **monoamine hypothesis** of depression, first proposed in the 1960s. This hypothesis suggested that mood disorders result from **deficiencies or imbalances in key neurotransmitters**.[89] The chemical imbalance idea was simple: low serotonin causes depressive symptoms, and selective serotonin reuptake inhibitors (SSRIs) like Prozac would fix that. But unfortunately, this explanation was nearly as reductive as saying that feelings of tiredness are *caused* by a "caffeine deficiency."

While coffee might be able to perk you up temporarily, it doesn't address why you're so tired in the first place. Similarly, antidepressants may improve mood and functioning for some, especially in the short term, but for many, there's a bigger story.

In their landmark 2022 umbrella review published in *Molecular Psychiatry*, Dr. Joanna Moncrieff and colleagues critically evaluated the **"serotonin hypothesis"** of depression—the idea that depression is caused by low serotonin levels in the brain.[90] They found **no consistent evidence** supporting the idea that depression is caused by low serotonin. Their findings challenged the biochemical explanation often used to justify the use of antidepressants, and called for a reevaluation of how mental health conditions are understood and treated.

Unsurprisingly, Dr. Joanna Moncrieff's findings received pushback, especially from psychiatrists with long-standing ties to the pharmaceutical industry. Moncrieff responded with a public statement, affirming that the widely accepted "chemical imbalance" theory was heavily promoted to the public, despite weak scientific backing. She referred to surveys that 85–90% of people in Western countries still believe depression is caused by a chemical imbalance—something that is not based in research and should no longer be communicated. As an alternative, she suggested rethinking how we understand antidepressants, noting they may work by creating a placebo effect or dulling emotional pain, rather than correcting any biological deficit.[91] Moncreiff's response is publicly available, and she is currently very active online in clearing up the confusion.

MULTIPLE PATHWAYS TO DEPRESSION

In any case, there is broad consensus that the causes of depression extend far beyond any one theory and include factors such as:

- Hormonal dysregulation
- Nutrition
- Environment
- Movement
- Inflammation
- Social connection / relationships
- Spiritual (or purpose-based) philosophies

My story is one of countless examples where the root causes of mental health struggles and whole-person solutions were unknowingly skipped over in favor of quick fixes. As the low-sugar decade dragged on, I found myself cycling through escalating doses of Prozac—20mg, then 30, 40, eventually 60. That's when the mental health rollercoaster really took off at full speed.

I often wonder—what if, instead of medication, I'd been guided toward real nourishment? A diet of whole foods, healthy fats, and quality proteins. Or how about nutrients in capsule form, like in the prison study? Or perhaps a prescription for movement, proven in some cases to rival antidepressants as we'll soon explore. None of these were even mentioned—and I'm not sure my doctor knew about their potential value in the 90's.

THE METABOLIC BREAKTHROUGH

In the spring of 2023, one of my podcast guests, renowned holistic psychiatrist Dr. Ellen Vora, introduced me to the work of Dr. Christopher L. Palmer, a psychiatrist at Harvard. I have so much respect for Dr. Vora's work and how she has been tirelessly researching holistic psychiatry and sharing it with the public for years now. When I asked her for resources on bipolar disorder so that I could better understand my own situation, Dr. Palmer was her first suggestion.

Dr. Palmer has made some big breakthroughs in the space of nutrition and brain health, especially when it comes to psychotic disorders.[92] Over the course of working with an extremely obese patient who was resistant to pharmaceuticals for his psychosis, Dr. Palmer immediately noticed mood and behavior improvements when his patient went on one specific type of diet. The patient had been suffering from extreme psychosis, and had been officially diagnosed with Schizophrenia. While there are no known, widely agreed upon cures for Schizophrenia in the medical field yet, there are medications widely used to manage symptoms. Unfortunately, many of those medications, namely antipsychotics, are notorious for having a host of side effects, oftentimes so severe that patients discontinue their meds. Common side effects of certain meds include dizziness and sedation, and long-term use can lead to significant health issues, including weight gain, type 2 diabetes, and metabolic syndrome.[93]

This was the beauty of Dr. Palmer's discovery—the Ketogenic diet managed to keep his patients' psychoses at bay without the unwanted side effects. The ketogenic diet is a high-fat, extremely low-carbohydrate nutrition plan that shifts the body into ketosis, where it burns fat for fuel instead of carbs.[94] This metabolic state can aid weight loss, improve energy, and potentially support certain health conditions like epilepsy and metabolic disorders. This nutrition plan *must* be created and supervised closely by a qualified practitioner.

As he's a scientist, Dr. Palmer tested his initial finding in the lab. He found a distinct connection between glucose metabolism, brain energy, and mental health outcomes in people with psychotic disorders. He has documented cases where patients with severe mental illnesses experienced significant improvements or remission of symptoms by following a ketogenic diet.

DR. PALMER'S BRAIN ENERGY THEORY

The Brain Energy Theory posits that mental disorders—including depression, anxiety, OCD, PTSD, bipolar disorder, and schizophrenia—are rooted in metabolic dysfunction. Specifically, impaired mitochondrial function and disrupted energy production in the brain lead to altered neural communication and compromised brain health.[95] By altering the body's metabolism to utilize ketones for energy instead of glucose, the ketogenic diet is one intervention aligned with the theory that *may* enhance mitochondrial function and energy production in brain cells.

Learning this, I immediately began to wonder if my own bipolar symptoms over the years were tied to my body and brain glucose metabolism. The idea that a targeted nutritional approach could address my symptoms was simply thrilling. Reflecting back over my dieting history, I realized quickly that my best periods of mental health were correlated with adhering to some of the lower-carb nutrition plans I had tried over the years.

When I discovered Dr. Palmer's work in the summer of 2023, I had been taking a hefty dose of prescription Seroquel (also known under the generic name Quetiapine), a dopamine blocking anti-psychotic, and was experiencing some *highly* undesirable side effects. To be honest, I felt like I was walking around in a chemical straitjacket. My motivation to get out of bed in the morning was gone. On a cognitive level, I knew I had a million and one incredible reasons to live, but *feeling* this motivation was completely and totally out of reach. Experiencing simple joys of daily life was out of reach. I cannot adequately articulate what it was like for me to be on such a high dose of dopamine blockers other than by telling you this: it was utterly miserable for me.

As I learned the hard way, Seroquel and other antipsychotics like it cause significant weight gain, sluggishness, and increased risk of metabolic syndrome and diabetes.[96] While they might be able to bring someone down from a manic high, that person can then land in a state of drug-induced sedation, like I did. My blood sugar was borderline Diabetic, and out of desperation, I had somehow accepted these drawbacks as part of the standard treatment I needed. I had accepted my suffering as an absolute, but finding the work of Dr. Palmer gave me a sense of hope I hadn't felt since before I was first diagnosed with bipolar at age 17.

STARTING KETO IN A TIME OF CRISIS

Despite my initial excitement, I procrastinated starting keto. It is a pretty restrictive diet, after all, and I wasn't sure that I needed any extra stress in my life. Travel plans, work commitments, and other excuses delayed me for months. Then, on October 7, 2023, everything shifted. A devastating mass terror attack targeted my country - a declaration of war - in what was the largest attack against Jewish people since the Holocaust. Our country was thrown into a state of absolute turmoil and ongoing war.

However, amid the fear, grief, immense loss, and uncertainty I was feeling, I also realized that I needed to prioritize my mental health above everything else to stay grounded, sane, and function at my best. In addition to the general fears of living in a war zone, I was also concerned that I'd start to lose sleep from all of the stress and wind up back in a psych ward. It would have been my eighth stay in a psych ward, but thankfully, what I implemented helped me to avoid this.

I began the ketogenic diet, expecting an uphill battle of sugar cravings, deprivation, and endless food prep. Instead, I was shocked: from the first day I started, my sugar cravings were gone, and for the first time in a long time, I felt largely satiated throughout the day. What I thought would be the hardest diet I'd ever tried turned out to be quite liberating, and it could not have come at a more critical moment in my life.

THE LIBERATION OF FINDING WHAT WORKS

Keto freed me from constant cravings for sweet foods. Even though I hadn't been indulging in sugary desserts regularly, I often battled cravings or a low-grade feeling of hunger, even after meals. On keto, those cravings vanished.

After about six months on keto, my body signaled it was time for a change. Under the guidance of an integrative doctor and my health coach, I transitioned to a nutrient-rich, modified keto-style diet emphasizing protein, fiber, moderately low healthy carbohydrates, and healthy fats. This approach has worked beautifully for me ever since. It's sustainable, balanced, energizing and it supports my mental and physical health without feeling restrictive.

Food truly is medicine, but the prescription may look a little different for everyone.

In chapter 1, we mentioned that most experts agree that Keto and other strict diets are not the right plan for everyone, and for some (like me), they may be a good short-term option. However, this diet necessitates working with a qualified health practitioner to guide you and make sure you're staying in a healthy range of ketosis, using a blood or breath monitor regularly. Please seek qualified, professional supervision if you think it could be an right for you. Either way, the research on mental health and nutrition is evolving, and it's definitely something to keep an eye on.

GUT HEALING THROUGH REDUCING INFLAMMATION

Inflammation has become a buzzword in health conversations, often painted as the ultimate villain. But inflammation itself isn't inherently bad. It's the body's way of communicating—activating immune cells to protect and heal itself. Take exercise, for example: after a workout, inflammatory pathways are triggered to repair muscles and strengthen bones. This is *positive* inflammation, helping the body rebuild stronger.[97]

The problem arises when inflammation becomes chronic. When the body's pro-inflammatory and anti-inflammatory mechanisms fall out of balance, inflammation can spiral out of control, driving a host of issues—from heart disease and Alzheimer's to depression.[98]

Research has shown that inflammation plays a significant role in mental health. This is true even for mice: chronic gut inflammation can induce anxiety-like behavior in mice and alter central nervous system biochemistry.[99] The immune system and inflammatory pathways interact with the brain, influencing mood and mental health. Addressing inflammation through diet and lifestyle can support the body's natural healing processes and promote emotional resilience.

ANTI-INFLAMMATORY NUTRITION: A SIMPLE SHIFT TOWARD WELLNESS

One of the most effective ways to reduce inflammation and support mental health is through anti-inflammatory nutrition.[100] Yes, specific foods are removed from the plate to create this plan, but when done right, it isn't about deprivation—it's about abundance. Think of an assortment of vibrant, colorful vegetables and fruits, lean proteins, whole grains, legumes, and healthy fats, all working together to nourish your body and mind into a state of harmony.

Anti-inflammatory nutrition can be transformational for almost anyone if paired with adequate sleep, regular movement, and stress management. Let's explore what this shift looks like.

Anti-inflammatory eating centers on whole, nutritious foods—like leafy greens, colorful vegetables, nutritious proteins, healthy fats, and fermented foods—that help calm inflammation in the body. At the same time, it minimizes foods known to fuel inflammation, such as refined sugar, processed meats, unhealthy fats, and ultra-processed snacks. This way of eating supports gut health, brain function, and overall well-being. Here is a basic overview:

I. EAT WHOLE FOODS.

Opt for fresh, unprocessed, or minimally processed ingredients whenever possible. Stock up on colorful veggies and fruits and aim to add new colors and diversify your repertoire each week. Start with as many above ground veggies as possible, which are lower in starch. Add in some root veggies, like potato and sweet potato, and a variety of seasonal fruits. If you're shopping in a big grocery store, stick to the perimeters where the fresh, frozen, and refrigerated foods are found. *Remember this phrase: if God made it, eat it. If man made it, leave it.* If your food is not 100% whole, check the ingredients. Stick to foods with minimal ingredients that you can pronounce. Herbs and spices are a great nutritional addition, and with no downside!

2. START YOUR DAY WITH SOMETHING SAVORY.

Skip the muffin, waffle, or cereal, and opt for a high-protein, high fiber breakfast instead. Think out of the box - what hearty proteins do you enjoy eating? You could incorporate meat or eggs into your breakfast, rounding it out with a small portion of healthy carbs and plenty of veggies. This will serve to stabilize your energy and focus throughout the day, and best of all, it's an approach known to lessen cravings for sweets in the afternoon and evening.

3. ADD MORE FRESH PRODUCE.

Aim for a variety of colorful vegetables and low-sugar fruits. By incorporating one big colorful salad into your day, you can get a ton of colors (and nutrients) into your body. There are endless types of chop salads, green salads, salads incorporating last night's leftovers - your options are endless! (Time-saving tip: make extra salad and store it in the fridge *without* dressing for use throughout the week.) Make sure to incorporate a serving of healthy protein and fat to make sure you feel satiated. Drink plenty of water before and during your meal for greater feelings of fullness- what often feels like hunger is the body craving water.

4. REDUCE OR ELIMINATE PROCESSED FOODS AND DRINKS.

Replace packaged snacks with their super-food counterparts. Fresh berries, fruit slices, and a handful of nuts can go a long way. Veggies and healthy dips are a great option - hummus, tahina, or nut dips can add a few grams of protein and some healthy satiating fats to your snack. Smoothies are a great way to pack in nutrients on the go - I opt for a quality protein powder, fresh berries, and an organic vegan milk base, or water, to stay clear of unnecessary carbs or sugars. You can add in a handful of veggies - frozen zucchini adds a creamy element, surprisingly like a banana with far less sugar. There are other awesome smoothie additions you can use for extra protein - if you're doing dairy, a high-protein yogurt is an option. A vegan addition like dehydrated peanut powder adds some creamy peanut butter flavor without unnecessary calories.

5. HYDRATE CONSISTENTLY.

Begin your day with a glass of lemon or apple cider vinegar (acv) water and keep a full water bottle handy throughout the day. Treat yourself to a nice-looking water bottle that you'll enjoy bringing along with you and refilling on the go. Instead of sugary soda, try a can of sparkling water to replace it. I love coffee- while the research does point to a connection with caffeine and mental health symptoms, a pre-workout coffee gives me just the boost I need. (Remember, the goal is not perfection, but progress and functioning!) Green tea is an alternative that boasts several health benefits and provides the body with caffeine. If anxiety is one of your symptoms, you may want to experiment with lowering your caffeine, especially if it's not before exercise or if it's being consumed later in the day. Water or herbal tea—plain and simple, or with a slice of lemon—are good options to always have on hand. Grab yourself a gorgeous water bottle that makes you smile when you see it, and always keep it by your side.

6. HAVE AN "ADDITION" MINDSET.

Instead of obsessing over what you can't have, prioritize *adding* nutrient-rich foods. Over time, cravings for processed foods will naturally diminish. If you're really craving that processed snack, don't deprive yourself. Begin by ensuring your body is fully hydrated, drinking extra water, and doing deep breathing to relax your nervous system. Have a nutrient-dense, healthy meal or snack and see how you feel afterward.

Giving in to an occasional craving is not bad if it helps you feel less deprived, setting you up to have more discipline over the long term. If you do eat that treat, eat it mindfully. Allow yourself to eat slowly, notice the flavors, textures, and sensations involved in your eating experience. Sometimes, people (me included) notice that the treat wasn't all that satisfying in the end—it was the thought of the treat, not being able to have it, and other associations with that treat that created the craving in the first place. I used to like all kinds of things that I don't eat anymore - and don't miss - whatsoever. By following this process, the same thing may happen to you. The bottom line is to feed yourself with the healthy nutrients your body needs and be compassionate with yourself if you slip up. Ditch the guilt—this is a process, and lasting change takes repetition. Do it all with the self-love that you deserve!

7. INCORPORATE BASIC SUPPLEMENTATION.

The most recommended foundation for supplementing often includes a quality multivitamin, a high-quality probiotic, and omega-3 fatty acids from fish oil. Magnesium is another nutrient that tends to be low in modern diets, in part due to soil depletion. Some people choose to support their magnesium levels with Epsom salt baths, chelated supplements like magnesium glycinate, or topical magnesium gels. Another interesting supplement that has gained visibility for its potential efficacy in abating depression symptoms is Creatine Monohydrate.[101] Always consult with a qualified practitioner to make sure supplements are the right choice for you. For an individualized approach, you can have your bloodwork evaluated by your clinician who can also address your specific needs and tailor your plan accordingly.

8. INCORPORATE HEALTHY FATS.

Avocado, nuts, seeds, and olive oil are excellent choices to fuel your body and support brain health. Adding a moderate amount to your meals will slow the body's absorption of sugars from your foods and create more stability in your blood sugar. For cooking, choose avocado oil or another non-seed oil with a high smoke point—like ghee or coconut oil—as these oils are more stable at high temperatures and less likely to break down into harmful compounds compared to seed oils like canola, soybean, or corn oil, which are often ultra-processed and can contribute to inflammation.[102] As this information is catching on, there's a growing trend to label food items or even restaurants as "seed-oil free."

9. PRACTICE MINDFUL EATING.

Slow down, take a few deep breaths, and express gratitude before you begin a meal. Notice the nuances in tastes and textures of your food and allow yourself to chew slowly so that you will enjoy and then digest each bite optimally. By eating mindfully, you're priming your body to lower cravings.

10. BE KIND TO YOURSELF AND ENJOY THE PROCESS.

Celebrate your progress, however seemingly great or small, and listen to your body's signals as you transition to a more supportive way of eating.

INFLAMMATION ELIMINATION PROTOCOL

If you want to take your anti-inflammatory nutrition one step further, you can experiment with an elimination protocol. An elimination protocol can be empowering when approached with curiosity about the experience and the results. Start by removing common inflammatory culprits for 3-4 weeks, including gluten, dairy, refined sugar, processed foods, industrial seed oils, alcohol, and artificial additives.

Focus on vibrant, whole foods: load your plate with colorful vegetables, lean proteins like wild-caught fish and pasture-raised chicken, healthy fats from avocado and olive oil, and nourishing carbs like sweet potatoes and quinoa. Hydrate with water, herbal teas, and green smoothies packed with anti-inflammatory superfoods like spinach and berries. Keep it fun by experimenting with new recipes, like turmeric-spiced roasted veggies or chia pudding. At the end of the elimination phase, reintroduce foods one at a time to learn how your body truly thrives.

WHAT TO AVOID TO REDUCE GUT INFLAMMATION

Here's a more detailed overview of what you want to avoid so that you can heal the gut and reduce inflammation. The anti-inflammatory nutrition plan aims to reduce gut inflammation by avoiding certain agents that are known to contribute to it. These include:

1. **Processed Foods and Additives:** This includes artificial sweeteners such as aspartame and sucralose, which can disrupt gut microbiota balance. Preservatives, including sulfites and nitrates, as well as emulsifiers, can irritate the gut lining. Instead, opt for whole, fresh foods. Make sure you read the ingredients for any packaged products.

2. **Refined Sugars:** Sugar promotes *dysbiosis*, which is an imbalance in gut bacteria. As we've discussed, it can dysregulate blood sugar, promote cravings, and even create addiction-like behaviors. Be mindful of sugars in packaged foods: yogurts, sauces, and packaged soups are all culprits. For something sweet, opt for whole fruits, ideally berries, which are lower in sugar, and try not to consume sweet foods on an empty stomach.

3. **Industrial Seed Oils:** Skipping seed oils is increasingly becoming mainstream, and for a good reason. Seed oils include soybean, corn, sunflower, and canola oil. These oils promote inflammation when consumed excessively relative to omega-3 fatty acids. Instead, opt for extra virgin olive oil, avocado, coconut, ghee, grass-fed butter, macadamia nut, sesame, flaxseed, or walnut oil. Note that flaxseed oil and walnut oil shouldn't be cooked, because they are sensitive to heat and can oxidize,

losing nutritional value and potentially producing harmful compounds. Stay away from seed oils, as we've discussed. They're often used in packaged, processed foods.

4. **Alcohol:** Skipping wine, beer, and liquor is a great move to heal the gut. Heavy drinking damages the gut lining and increases permeability, aka "leaky gut." It also increases unhealthy inflammation.[103] Before we go any further, I'm not here to be the fun police; everyone's path is personal. The most important thing is tuning into what truly supports your well-being and helps you feel your best.

There's increasing evidence that even more moderate amounts of drinking pose health risks. Bottled alcohols may include an array of additives, preservatives, and chemicals, so you're doing your body a solid favor by skipping that drink. If you're into your alcohol, you may be disappointed here that there aren't great substitutes. I opt for tea or sparkling water, and make sure that I'm not hungry, which increases alcohol cravings.

As someone who genuinely enjoyed drinking in my younger years, I've come to realize that it wasn't the alcohol itself that made those moments special—it was the connection, the laughter, the music, and the atmosphere. It was also the savvy marketing campaigns up and down Sunset Boulevard, painting a picture of freedom, enjoyment, and connection that I, like so many others, bought into without a second thought.

The good news? All of those benefits are possible without a drink in hand—and often even more enjoyable with full presence and energy.

If you're in social environments where alcohol is prevalent, think about alternative social activities that you can do to keep you connected but away from this toxin while you're adhering to anti-inflammation nutrition. If you are absolutely set on having that glass of wine, drink water and replenish your body with nutrients first so that you'll be more inclined to enjoy the taste of your beverage rather than feel tempted to gulp it down for thirst or hunger quenching.

5. **Gluten:** If you're sensitive to gluten or you have a condition like celiac disease, gluten, a protein found in certain grains, can trigger an inflammatory response in the gut. Another potential issue with grains is that store-bought breads may contain preservatives and additives, and the flour in those

loaves may have been grown with pesticides or genetic modification. You can support your gut healing by skipping wheat, barley, malt, bulgur, farro, spelt, semolina, and couscous. Instead, focus on eating a wide variety of veggies. By way of carby sides, you can go for alternatives such as rice, quinoa, cauliflower, zucchini, sweet potato, potato, and squash.

6. **Dairy:** Certain people may react to casein or lactose in dairy, causing inflammation and digestive issues. By way of most foods, you can find a non-dairy alternative. There are lots of milk substitutes on the market these days. Choices include almond, hemp, coconut, cashew, and others. Be sure to choose organic when possible and opt for the ones with fewer ingredients and no additives, sugar, or preservatives.

After eliminating the above six foods over the course of a **3–4 week inflammation elimination diet,** the reintroduction phase begins. This can help you identify food sensitivities by slowly adding back foods one at a time. Start by checking in with your body and observing what kind of changes you notice, especially by way of your mood and energy. Next, introduce **one food type,** and observe how you feel for at least **2–3 days. Look out for** any common reactions like bloating, headaches, fatigue, joint pain, or skin changes. If no symptoms occur, the food is likely safe to eat; if symptoms return, remove the food again. Following the same process, you can keep a food journal to track reactions and introduce new foods gradually. This approach helps pinpoint any possible inflammatory triggers and supports your long-term gut health. If you need extra support in the process, you may want to consider working with a qualified health provider.

REDEFINING NUTRITION FOR LONG-TERM HEALTH

Nutrition is the foundation of health, including mental health, but it's not just about *what* you eat. It's about creating a lifestyle that supports your overall well-being. Remember, food fuels your body, impacts your mood, and supports thriving overall.

You don't need to be perfect; this isn't about following a rigid set of rules forever. It's about learning to understand what your body and mind need in order to thrive. It's about nourishing yourself in a way that feels good, both physically and emotionally. With small, consistent changes, you'll discover that food isn't just fuel—it's medicine and can transform your life and gut health.

CHAPTER 8 SUMMARY

KEY CONCEPTS

1. **There's a dopamine vs. serotonin dilemma.** The overconsumption of sugar fuels dopamine-driven pleasure-seeking behavior, which can lead to addiction, while serotonin, the neurotransmitter linked to long-term happiness, thrives on balanced nutrition and meaningful social connections.

2. **Understand the gut-brain connection.** A healthy gut microbiome plays a crucial role in mental well-being, as the majority of serotonin is produced in the gut, highlighting the importance of consuming fiber-rich and whole foods over processed ones.

3. **Use nutrition as medicine.** Scientific evidence supports using food to support mental health, with anti-inflammatory diets, nutrient-dense whole foods, and balanced macronutrient intake helping to reduce inflammation, regulate mood, and improve overall health outcomes.

QUESTIONS

1. How can having an "addition" mindset help you practice self-compassion on this journey toward gut and mental health? What small steps can you add to your daily routine to nourish your body?

2. What is your "why" for reducing gut inflammation? Write down all your desired results (improved mood, more energy, less fatigue, etc.) and keep them where you can refer to them often for motivation.

3. How have you previously defined *pleasure* and *happiness*? How have your thoughts on these concepts changed, if at all, when you consider your mental well-being?

CHAPTER 9

THE REST REVOLUTION

*"Sleep is a sacred surrender, a daily
trust fall into the hands of healing."*

—unknown

As a high school senior in 1998, I felt invincible. Prozac had given me a surge of energy, and even though I had been dealing with on-and-off depression symptoms, I was thriving academically and socially. Sleep began to feel like an optional activity— a luxury I didn't think I needed— I'd stay up past midnight, rise with the sun, and still feel wired for the day.

What I didn't realize then—and what we know more clearly now—is that SSRIs like Prozac can trigger manic or hypomanic episodes in some people.[104] But at 17, I had no idea what mania even was… although it was beginning to creep into my life.

One sunny Sunday that April, full of energy, I decided to bike 18 miles to visit some friends in a nearby beach town. When I arrived, high on adrenaline, I found my friends skateboarding—something I'd never really done before. Seconds later, I was flying down a hill far too steep for me… and I crashed, breaking my left leg in two places.

Whether it was a lack of sleep or too much Prozac running through my veins and inspiring impulsivity, I was pushing my limits too hard that day. I spent the next several weeks with my left foot in a cast.

When the end of June rolled around, the cast was removed, but the metal hardware inside my foot was still in place. On yet another sunny afternoon, now in July, I boarded a plane to Europe with my youth group, naively unaware of the havoc this long flight could wreak on my post-surgery body.

SLEEP LOSS AND SPIRALING INTO MANIA

An hour into the flight, my foot began to swell. Pain consumed me, and sleeping became impossible. Over the next three days, as we moved from Rome to Prague to Israel, the lack of sleep, physical agony, and mounting stress brought me to the edge of what my body and mind could handle. By the time we reached Israel, my mind was slipping. Bright white light fractured into rainbows, reality blurred, and I found myself dazed and detached. I was hallucinating. I was rushed to the emergency room, and the trip organizers insisted I return home.

A MOMENT OF CLARITY AMID CHAOS

Before leaving, one of our trip counselors drove me to see the Western Wall. The experience, though fragmented in my memory, was profound in its impact. I stood gazing at the Temple Mount, a symbol of over 3,000 years of history, feeling a deep connection to my ancestors. The white stone shimmered with rainbow light, and despite my altered state, I felt a profound clarity: this was an epicenter of ancient spiritual and ethical foundations that had shaped our world in huge ways. This moment stayed with me as I returned home, grappling with sleeplessness and confusion.

Sitting on my parents' balcony the first morning back, I ate a slice of cantaloupe. The simple act of tasting its sweet, juicy flesh in the summer sun became a revelation. I realized that life's smallest joys could hold infinite beauty if I leaned into them. Colors were brighter and crisper. Flavors were rich and nuanced. I was in and out of experiencing hallucinations that included profound micro-moments of bliss. But these hallucinations were also scary, and potentially dangerous, leading to the unfortunate moment of receiving a diagnosis and prescriptions, robbing me of blissful sensations for years to come. I paid a very high price for the sleepless nights on my summer trip.

THE DANGER OF SLEEP DEPRIVATION

In today's fast-paced world, sleep often takes a backseat to the endless to-do lists and digital distractions. Most people are sleep-deprived, missing out on the mental health benefits of quality sleep. However, sleep and mental health are critically connected.

Sleep loss is so hazardous to our health that extended sleep deprivation studies are considered unethical. The research we *do* have around sleep reveals stark consequences. Within 24 to 48 hours without sleep, most people experience symptoms of anxiety, irritability, and disorientation. By 72 to 90 hours, hallucinations, delusions, and a psychotic-like state are common. A 2018 study concluded that sleep deprivation progressively leads to "psychotic symptoms," with normal sleep often resolving these effects—but not always.[105]

Even without extreme deprivation, poor sleep is also closely linked to mental health symptoms, including depression, anxiety, and suicidal ideation. Sleep deprivation doesn't just take a toll on your mind; it can wreak havoc on the body, and let's face it: walking around rested makes life a lot more pleasant.

SLEEP AND STRESS

How much are people sleeping these days, really? In 1942, over 60% of US adults reported sleeping 8 or more hours per night, with only 3% sleeping 5 hours or fewer. By 2023, only 26% remained in the 8 or more range, while 20% were sleeping 5 hours or fewer.[106] Over the same period, we've seen exponential growth of technology, allowing (or *obligating*) people to work from home. Most of today's jobs didn't even exist in the 1940s. When we were kids in the 80s, our parents would go on vacations, and the only way they could work was by sending a fax. Today, many employed and self-employed adults work from laptops and smartphones, which can easily blur the lines between work, leisure, and even *sleep* time.

INVISIBLE LABOR AND STRESS IN THE HOME

We can also examine the phenomenon of shifting gender roles to understand why home and child-rearing responsibilities may be a source of added stress for some. If you're a woman who grew up with a stay-at-home mom taking on most of the domestic roles and is now trying to balance work and home responsibilities, are you sharing those responsibilities with a partner, or are you trying to do it all?

A 2024 article in *The Atlantic* called "Put Down the Vacuum" sheds insight on how "mothers spend twice as much time as fathers 'on the essential and unpaid work' of taking care of kids and the home, and that women spend more time on this than men, regardless of parental and relationship status."[107] The author also notes that **women's cortisol levels rise more than their male counterparts' when their home spaces are out of order.**

If you're reading this and identifying with feeling stressed by a mess, it's worth evaluating what you can do to change things up. *The Atlantic* article hints at a few ideas to lighten your load: share responsibilities, simplify your home space to minimize your workload, order groceries online, outsource help if you can, buy a robot vacuum, or delegate tasks to other people in your home so that you can feel calmer in your space.

Of course, it's important to recognize that access to these solutions often reflects a level of privilege—not every woman or family has the same resources or support. The ability to outsource help, order groceries online, or hire cleaning services isn't always available.

No matter your current circumstances, there are empowering steps you can take. Whether it's establishing a clearer division of labor at home, setting boundaries around your time, or devising creative, low-cost solutions to minimize stress, the key is finding what works for *you*.

I've found that having drawers or closets (covered spaces) instead of open shelves is one quick fix if I need to put things away in a pinch. The space looks organized, and when I have a few extra minutes on hand, I can come back to the space and tidy it up. With compassion and intention, we can all take meaningful steps to create more ease in our environments.

As someone who has struggled with wanting everything to look "just so" in my home over the years, I've learned to speak to myself with self-compassion and remind myself that a little clutter or a pile of dishes in the sink doesn't define me or my worth as a mom and wife. It simply means that life is busy, my home is lived in, and we all have a lot going on, which is a beautiful thing. Best of all, feeling calmer in our home spaces can be huge by way of shifting from work mode into rest mode, and getting a healthy night's sleep. One of my friends, a busy mom of six young children always reminds me, "a house is not a museum."

We need to prioritize our sleep as a non-negotiable. Have an open conversation with the people you live with about dividing chores and drop the guilt about all the things you're not able to get done (or don't want to get done) on any given day. Now, it's possible that your to-do list is providing you with satisfaction and a quality short-term dopamine hit that you don't want to sacrifice for the sake of sleep. However, by internalizing the importance of sleep, you can literally add it to your to-do list and be sure to put it at the top when you do.

WHY SLEEP MATTERS

I learned the hard way that sleep isn't a luxury; it's a non-negotiable foundation of health. In a world where we're marketed productivity over rest, we need to flip the script and call out the nonsense. By understanding the science of sleep and making intentional changes, you can reclaim this vital pillar of health.

Sleep is the cornerstone of physical and mental health. Without it, the body and mind falter. Consistent sleep patterns are strongly correlated with improved mental health, cognitive functioning, and reduced risks of chronic conditions. A 2023 study of more than 88,000 people's sleep data over the course of seven years found that individuals with irregular sleep-wake patterns had higher mortality risks.[108] This underscores the importance of not only *time asleep* but also *what* time you go to sleep and wake up each day, and trying to create consistency around those times.

Your physiology and feelings are directly impacted by what's around and inside of you at any given moment. It's what you eat, drink, your sleep habits, the air you breathe, how you move, and the light you absorb. It's how your body processes energy, eliminates toxins, and interacts with your environment. Habits like consistent sleep, regular movement, and soaking up morning sunlight are simple yet powerful ways to optimize your mental and physical health. And let's not forget the fun stuff, which we'll also get into—like relaxing under infrared light, sipping a cozy tea, or walking barefoot in the grass. These moments of joy and connection with nature can also profoundly impact your physiology.

Your bedtime is another important variable in the context of your overall mental health. A 2024 study of 73,000 people in the UK found that individuals who went to sleep the latest had a **20-40% higher risk** of being diagnosed with a mental health disorder.[109] The researchers tested the possibility that poor mental health was causing the later bedtime but found that even among those night owls with no previous diagnosis, **night owls who went to bed *and* woke up later were still the most prone to receiving diagnoses later on.**

NATURAL LIGHT CYCLES

We can learn from preindustrial societies that align sleep with natural light cycles and report having better mental health states, reinforcing that our bodies thrive when synced with nature's rhythms. Three pre-industrial societies have been the subjects of academic research on sleep: the Hadza of Tanzania, the San of Namibia, and the **Tsimané** of the Bolivian Amazon.[110] Living without electricity, these groups align their sleep with natural light and temperature cycles. Insomnia is rare in these groups, and the study found no indicators of poor mental health. All three societies showed similar sleep schedules, with average durations between 5.7 and 7.1 hours, which is similar to people in modern societies.

The main difference between these three preindustrial societies and their modern counterparts is their earlier sleep schedules. Bedtimes average 3.3 hours after sunset, and wake times are before or around sunrise. It's also interesting that for the groups living in regions experiencing shorter winters, the average sleep duration was over fifty minutes more during the darker season.

Although we're not living in these preindustrial societies, we *can* choose to make upgrades that more closely align our sleep with nature. Small, intentional changes can lead to big improvements with sleep. Here are a few foundational strategies to help you optimize your sleep:

MORNING RITUALS TO SUPPORT NIGHTLY REST

- **Absorb Natural Light:** Spend time outside in the morning without sunglasses. This exposure sets your body's internal clock, helping it release melatonin 14-16 hours later.

- **Stay Active:** Moving your body during the day supports deeper, more restorative sleep at night.

EVENING WIND-DOWN STRATEGIES

- **Limit Artificial Light:** Reduce screen time and dim the lights in your home in the evening. Consider using blue-light-blocking glasses after sunset.

- **Go Sunset Gazing:** Go outside during sunset time, without sunglasses, for at least ten minutes. Don't look directly at the sun; you can look at the sky. Let yourself enjoy this healthy ritual.

- **Evening Meal:** Eat a high-quality carbohydrate along with your *early* evening meal to promote restfulness.

- **Create a Calming Environment:** Keep your bedroom free of clutter, work materials, and any visual or auditory stressors.

- **Control Temperature and Light:** Ensure your room is cool, dark, and quiet. Use blackout curtains, eye masks, and earplugs if needed. Cover up any bright lights coming from air conditioners, clocks, etc.

BEDTIME RITUALS FOR DEEP SLEEP

- **Go to Bed Earlier:** Deep sleep primarily occurs early, so an earlier bedtime supports the body's most restorative processes.

- **Use a Sleep Tracker:** Devices like smartwatches can provide valuable insights into your sleep patterns, motivating you to stick to healthier routines.

Tracking my sleep revealed something fascinating: most of my deep sleep happens before midnight. That simple insight, delivered by a sleep tracking device, completely shifted how I approach bedtime. It turned rest into a kind of game—one where the reward is better mood, clearer thinking, and more energy. While there's no universal formula for perfect sleep, the research is clear on the power of consistency and timing.

THE POWER OF CONSISTENT SLEEP

For me, consistent, high-quality sleep isn't just a nice-to-have—it's a cornerstone of my self-care. I'll be honest: I regularly turn down evening invites. Not because I don't enjoy a good night out, but because I've come to understand how essential it is to protect this boundary for my well-being. On occasion—once or twice a month—I'll make space for a night out, but I try to be mindful of the environment. I steer clear of synthetic spaces filled with loud music and bright screens, knowing how much they can throw off my rhythm. It's not about restriction—it's about aligning choices with what helps me feel my best.

I've found that filling my days with meaningful social connection helps me wind down more easily at night—and keeps me from overstimulating my nervous system after dark. I'm a big fan of scheduling and time-blocking to make room for focused work, movement, and things that nourish me. Of course, I'm not suggesting you skip out on evening plans altogether—connection is essential to our well-being. But it can be powerful to notice what kinds of nighttime activities actually leave you feeling your best the next day. It's worth experimenting with what works for your rhythm, so you can align your evenings with the kind of energy you want to carry forward. Remember that you are the CEO of your health, your time, and your life. Just because you've always done things a certain way doesn't mean there aren't infinite other options available, some of which may pleasantly surprise you for their added value.

Let's dive deeper into how you can harness the power of sleep to transform your well-being. Whether you're struggling to fall asleep, stay asleep, or feel rested, there are solutions.

TRANSITIONING FROM PRODUCTIVITY TO REST: A VITAL SLEEP STRATEGY

One of the most challenging aspects of falling asleep is shifting from productivity mode to rest mode. For anyone who experiences extreme moods or heightened emotional states, this transition can feel especially elusive. Making intentional adjustments to reframe evenings as wind-down time, and creating a restful environment has worked wonders for me.

The first step is becoming extremely selective about how you spend your evenings, and remove any unnecessary stimulation that may be overly activating and keep you awake far past bedtime. Think about this as reallocating activities that *energizes* you to the daytime, and schedule activities in the evenings that are more conducive to *relaxation*.

Invited to dinner? How about opting for lunch instead? While you can allow yourself some flexibility with nights, especially if sleep is not a major issue for you, be mindful about how late you're staying out, and the stimuli in your environment. Activating stimuli can make you feel awake even well after you're back home and in bed but still experiencing the high from all the action. Starting and ending your evenings earlier can also make a big difference. Minimizing nighttime obligations may feel like a limit to your social life, but the trade-off can be well worth it.

REFRAMING REST AS A PRIORITY

I once described my early bedtime routine to a therapist, wondering out loud why I had to be so restricted. I had labeled this my "special need," feeling a pang of self-pity that I had to miss out on many opportunities. Her response was unexpected: "Serious athletes and high performers are also mindful about sleep." She's right. Just as athletes prioritize their recovery to perform at their best, prioritizing sleep is a cornerstone of overall health and well-being, especially for anyone navigating unwanted mental health-related symptoms.

Reframing rest as essential rather than optional has allowed me to embrace my evening routine without guilt. I no longer see it as a limitation but as a deliberate choice to honor my body and mind. And it feels amazing to feel amazing! As with all the upgrades, try this one on for size, and see how adjusting your daily routines to happen earlier affects your mood and energy levels. The more you notice positive effects from an upgrade, the more motivated you'll be to sustain it!

IMPLEMENTING BETTER SLEEP WITH THE ECHO METHOD

Using the ECHO method—Education, Curiosity, Healing, and Observation—you can create your own strategy for transitioning into rest mode and improving your sleep patterns. Here's how:

I. EDUCATION

- Learn about the impact of light, movement, and evening habits on your sleep cycle. Understand how prioritizing rest can transform your mental and physical health.

- Reflect on calming evening activities like walking outdoors, having a sauna, dimming your lights indoors, lighting candles, or other soothing activities that complement the energy of rest.

2. CURIOSITY

- Get curious about the benefits of making various upgrades. What happens if you dim your lights an hour earlier or avoid screens before bed? How will you experience this environment, and what other changes will take place when the mood shifts in your home (or your bedroom)?

3. HEALING

- Implement the upgrades that resonate with you the most, first. Start small and build a routine that feels manageable and restorative.

- Allow yourself to experience the potential energy shifts in your mind and body.

4. OBSERVATION

- Track your sleep patterns and mood changes. Use a sleep tracker or journal to note how adjustments affect your overall well-being.

- Reflect on what's most supportive, and refine your routine over time, celebrating the improvements you see.

BUILD YOUR SLEEP FOUNDATION TO THRIVE

Transitioning from productivity to rest mode is not always easy, but it's a skill you can cultivate with intention and patience. Applying the ECHO method will create a personalized evening routine that supports restful, rejuvenating sleep.

Remember, prioritizing sleep isn't just about logging hours in bed—it's about creating an environment and mindset that allows your body to recover and your mind to recharge. Like an athlete preparing for peak performance, you're building a foundation for your entire being to thrive! Your sleep journey starts tonight. You deserve to wake up feeling refreshed, restored, and ready to take on the day.

CHAPTER 9 SUMMARY

KEY CONCEPTS

1. **Sleep deprivation can have detrimental effects.** Lack of sleep significantly impacts mental health, with studies showing that prolonged sleep deprivation can induce symptoms of anxiety, hallucinations, and cognitive decline, while even moderate sleep loss increases the risk of depression, bipolar disorder, and schizophrenia.

2. **Modern sleep challenges play a part in mental health.** Sleep quality has declined over the decades due to stress, artificial light, and shifting societal roles, with women disproportionately affected by sleep deprivation, highlighting the need to set boundaries and prioritize rest.

3. **Optimize sleep for well-being.** Establishing consistent sleep routines, aligning with natural light cycles, and creating an evening wind-down routine can enhance both mental and physical health, reinforcing that sleep is not a luxury but a necessity for thriving.

QUESTIONS

1. **What are your lowest hanging fruits when it comes to improving your sleep routine?** Take a few moments to reflect on the habits or patterns that, if shifted, could help you feel more rested and restored. Consider writing

them down and ranking them in order of what feels most important or impactful to start with. Small changes can lead to big transformations.

2. Bringing awareness to the potential sources of stress in your environment is a powerful step. When you name what's on your mind, you create space to gently address it and move toward more restful nights. What shifts feel within reach for you in this moment?

3. Are you sharing responsibilities with a partner or roommate, or are you trying to do it all? Would it be at all possible to divide up labor or reorganize your schedule so that you can reprioritize sleep health?

4. What are some realistic, calming rituals that you can incorporate into your evening to promote a feeling of winding down and settling into sleep?

CHAPTER 10

MOVING FORWARD

*"You put your whole self in… and
you shake it all about."*

—*The Hokey Pokey*

I discovered the transformational power of movement out of sheer desperation. It was 1999, and I had moved back into my parents' house after having to leave university and losing my academic scholarship. I was weighed down—literally and figuratively—by the physical and emotional effects of Lithium.

I'd gained over 20 pounds since beginning treatment, and on top of this I felt disconnected from myself, emotionless, and hopeless about the future. My older brother, a fitness enthusiast, personal trainer, and budding bodybuilder at the time, used to repeat this mantra to me, any time he noticed I was looking remotely receptive: "Get in the best shape of your life, and everything else will follow." For a while, I resisted his invitations to join him at the gym, convinced that he didn't understand my situation, also secretly wondering if I was abnormally beyond help. But eventually, his relentlessness got through to me, and I decided to give it a shot.

THE TRANSFORMATIVE POWER OF EXERCISE

My brother guided me through the basics of strength training: heart rate, shoulder retraction, core engagement, weights, and cardio. Working with him was a precious gift that keeps giving, nearly thirty years later.

Recruiting someone to guide you, who believes in your potential to thrive can work absolute wonders. For me, the gym transformed from a foreign land into a personal sanctuary where I can focus on making an effort and seeing tangible results in my workouts. I recognize that having access to a personal trainer at that time in my life was a gift and a privilege—not everyone has that kind of support readily available. The empowering news is that today, expert guidance is more accessible than ever. Whether or not a trainer is in the cards for you, there's a wealth of high-quality, guided workouts available online—many of them completely free—so you can begin building strength and momentum on your own terms.

Back in 1999, it only took a few weeks before I noticed changes—not just in my body, but in my mind. The post-workout endorphin rush lifted my mood, and the sense of accomplishment countered the isolation and shame I had been feeling after a failed freshman year of university.

Fitness and academics became my lifelines. I adhered to a high-protein, high fiber and nutrient dense meal plan, worked out daily, and even became a certified spinning instructor to hold myself accountable to show up to the gym and exercise. By prioritizing movement, I reclaimed vital aspects of my mental health and began to rebuild my life.

MOVEMENT IS NOT A LUXURY

Over the years, life has become increasingly busy. Between work, parenting four children, moving across the world, and studying for three university degrees, I've fallen in and out of various exercise routines. However, one thing has become abundantly clear: my best years are the ones when I move consistently. Movement isn't a luxury; it's a necessity, especially in relation to mental health.

In recent years, I've become very consistent with daily movement. It's one of the most reliable tools I have for boosting mood, sustaining energy, and supporting overall well-being. Just an hour of movement—a little over 4% of the day—can have a powerful impact on the remaining 95%. I didn't always have this consistency; it has taken time and some thoughtful strategy to figure out what actually works. Next, I'll walk you through what helped me get here.

MOVEMENT AND DEPRESSIVE SYMPTOMS

When it comes to the mental health effects of movement, the research is both clear and astounding: movement is at least as effective as antidepressants in reducing non-severe depressive symptoms. A 2022 study in the *British Journal of Sports Medicine* analyzed 41 studies of over 2,200 participants and confirmed what many have long suspected: **"Exercise is an efficacious treatment option for reducing depressive symptoms for individuals with depression."**[111] The catch, of course, is that movement requires time and effort exceeding what is required to swallow pills. Like taking pills, it also requires consistency.

FINDING THE RIGHT KIND OF MOVEMENT

There's no one-size-fits-all approach to exercise, and the key is finding activities that resonate with you. In 2022, a systematic review and network meta-analysis published in *Sports Medicine – Open* looked at 117 randomized controlled trials involving over 6,400 participants to explore how different forms of exercise support mental health.[112] The results were pretty eye-opening: **multimodal exercise programs**—those that mix different types of movement—came out on top for easing depressive symptoms and the negative symptoms of schizophrenia.

Resistance training stood out as particularly helpful for **anxiety**, while **mind-body practices** like yoga and tai chi were most effective for **PTSD symptoms**. The takeaway? When it comes to movement, one size doesn't fit all. Matching the type of exercise to your unique mental health needs can make all the difference.

Here's a breakdown of different types of movement and their mental health benefits:

CARDIO (AEROBIC EXERCISE)

- **Examples:** Running, jogging, biking, swimming

- **Benefits:** Boosts endorphins and serotonin, reduces symptoms of depression and anxiety, and improves mood with around 30 minutes of moderate intensity.

STRENGTH TRAINING (GENERALLY ANAEROBIC)

- **Examples:** Weightlifting, bodyweight exercises, resistance bands

- **Benefits:** Enhances self-esteem, reduces depression symptoms, and supports cognitive function. Improves bone density, builds muscle, builds confidence, and supports longevity.

Here's something remarkable: having more muscle helps regulate blood sugar by acting as a major site for glucose disposal, which can improve insulin sensitivity and support metabolic health. In fact, higher muscle mass is associated with better metabolic function overall and a decreased risk for type 2 diabetes.[113] But the impact doesn't stop there—metabolic health and mental health are deeply intertwined. As Dr. Casey Means explains in *Good Energy*, metabolic dysfunction—especially blood sugar instability—is one of the most overlooked root causes of mood swings, anxiety, and even depression.[114] Supporting muscle and metabolic health isn't just about physical vitality—it's a key pillar of emotional well-being, too.

On a personal note, I'll tell you that this one has made me feel my *absolute best* over the years. I've learned to look forward to and enjoy my strength training workouts. What I also love about it is its versatility for people with injuries or limitations. There are so many variations of strength training exercises that it's not hard to work around injuries.

HEART RATE RECOMMENDATION

It's recommended to engage in moderate activity for at least 150 minutes per week, which has also been proven effective as an antidepressant for mood. The moderate range is one in which you keep your heart rate at 60-70% of your calculated maximum. Dr. Means, an expert in metabolic health, provides the number 64% of MHR as the specific target.[115] To calculate your ideal moderate heart rate recommendation, do the following:

1. **Find your Max Heart Rate (MHR):** subtract your age from 220.

2. Multiply this number by .64; the result is your ideal moderate training heart rate range.

You might not always break a sweat or get your heart rate into the moderate zone with slower movement practices, but that doesn't mean they're not incredibly powerful. A lot of people find a deep sense of grounding and well-being through practices like **yoga, tai chi, and qigong**.

Yoga blends mindful movement with breath and presence, helping to calm the nervous system, reduce stress, and support emotional balance. Tai chi and qigong use slow, intentional motions to promote relaxation and mental clarity, making them beautiful tools for restoring both body and mind.

Full disclosure—while I aspire to bring more slow forms of movement into my routine, I haven't done it yet. I'm sharing this with you because **I know there's a lot to take in here, and I want to keep it real: this journey isn't about doing it all perfectly.** It's about tuning in to what feels right for you, honoring your preferences, and making progress in a way that's sustainable and supportive.

MUSIC AND NATURE WITH MOVEMENT

Admittedly, yoga and tai chi aren't my thing (yet), but I do love a good mindful walk or hike, especially green ones, in nature. If you're moving steadily, going up hills, or wearing a weighted vest or backpack, you can reap the benefits of nature and get into your ideal moderate heart rate zone. This therapeutic combo can reduce stress, inspire creativity, and boost mood. Enjoy your green hikes and walks with some company for an added social benefit.

Dancing is another way to reap the therapeutic benefits of exercise. Combined with music and social interaction, dance can enhance mood, reduce anxiety, and even improve memory. World-renowned psychiatrist Dr. James Gordon discusses a particularly therapeutic form of dance in his groundbreaking book about post-traumatic growth, *The Transformation*.[116] I love how this simple practice can have such profound benefits. Dr. Gordon has helped countless people around the world recover from trauma, including populations affected by war. It's a tangible approach to fostering healing and resilience at almost any moment.

"Shaking and Dancing" is an expressive meditation technique designed to alleviate the physiological impacts of trauma. It's a trauma-informed movement method which involves vigorously shaking the body to let go of tension and disrupt the body's stress response. This is followed by free-form dancing to restore balance and promote relaxation. What I love so much about this technique is its accessibility.

MAKING MOVEMENT A HABIT

The hardest part of exercise is often just starting. As with riding a bike, in the beginning, it can feel difficult and wobbly, but once you get going, there's a lot of momentum and enjoyment. Here are some strategies to help you get moving and stay consistent:

1. START SMALL.

Start with 10 minutes a day to build momentum and end on a high note. Work up gradually and as you begin to feel more motivated. Every time you work out when you don't want to, you're training your brain and body to be more resilient and growing a fundamental region in your brain, your **anterior mid-cingulate cortex (AMCC)**, that regulates willpower.[117]

2. FIND ACCOUNTABILITY.

Partner with a friend, join a class in person or online, or work with a trainer. One caveat about partnering with a friend for accountability is that you don't want to be *relying* on someone else to show up so that you can work out. You can make plans to meet a friend to exercise or walk but take it upon yourself to do the movement even if your workout buddy cancels.

One way to stay accountable to your fitness goals is by becoming an instructor, especially if you're committed to making a particular movement type a part of your lifestyle in the long run. In the summer of 1999, becoming a spin instructor kept me accountable in a huge way - no longer could I hit the snooze button on the alarm and skip spin class, because I had to show up and teach! It got me into the gym and moving multiple times per week, which was invaluable for consistency.

I get it—it's not always realistic to just flip a switch and "become the instructor." During a rough patch in my mental health journey in later years, I knew I needed some kind of accountability, but I didn't have the energy or motivation to even get to the gym. Instead, I got creative. I reached out to a few friends and asked if they'd take turns coming over, alternating mornings, to do simple workouts with me on my balcony. I told them in advance, "Come over no matter what—even if I text you not to." It wasn't about doing a perfect workout—this was about getting out of bed in the morning during a difficult time, and making my best attempt to feel better.

3. COMBINE MOVEMENT WITH JOY.

Dance or workout to your favorite songs, hike in a beautiful location, or try a sport you've always wanted to explore. By stacking an enjoyable habit with movement, you're creating a positive association, which can go a long way in motivating you to continue and even look forward to your sessions.

Another way to combine movement with joy is by investing in workout clothes you love that make you feel comfortable. They don't have to be expensive, and you only need a few sets to start. Sometimes, simply putting them on can be enough to give you a boost of joy and motivation. Bright colors can even give you a dopamine boost before you start moving, enhancing the good vibes from your workout. Feeling fabulous can set the tone for an energizing session.

4. SET A ROUTINE.

Schedule movement as if it's a crucial work appointment. Block exercise into your calendar to ensure that nothing else gets in the way.

5. TRACK YOUR PROGRESS.

Use a fitness tracker or journal to celebrate milestones. Tracking your progress can motivate you to work out, making movement doubly satisfying. Write down your starting baseline metrics—weights, repetitions, distances, or times. Tracking your progress gives your brain a hit of feel-good hormones when you see improvement, and immediately after you write it down. This provides the same satisfaction as crossing something off your to-do list. I love jotting down my workouts with fun-colored pens and making tally marks for each set, à la Arnold Schwarzenegger, though I stick to a standard 3–5 sets, not Arnold's 25. Unless you're training to become the next Hercules, 3-5 sets per strength exercise should do the trick.

IMPLEMENTING MOVEMENT WITH THE ECHO METHOD

Let's apply the ECHO method—Education, Curiosity, Healing, Observation—to integrate movement into your routine:

1. **Education:** Learn about the mental health benefits of exercise and explore the types of movement that resonate with you. Learn with a trainer or by watching online videos created by professionals to give you the tools, strategies, and proper form that you need to partake in your chosen movement type.

2. **Curiosity:** Experiment with different activities that promote your desired benefits. Approach movement as an adventure. Ask yourself how you're feeling as you move; connect with your breath, and imagine that each ounce of effort will pay off with benefits for your body and mind.

3. **Healing:** Be mindful of your progress. Are your muscles feeling sore? Are you approaching daily activities with more energy? Are you craving healthier foods and more water? Focus on how the exercise makes you feel both during your sessions and in the days afterward.

4. **Observation:** Reflect on changes in your mood, energy, and outlook. Adjust your routine based on what feels best for you and provides you with the most benefit. Incorporate the types of movement that are the most additive to your life.

CELEBRATE YOUR PROGRESS

Instead of focusing on external outcomes like changes in your physique, celebrate the effort and progress in your more immediate control. Adding more weight to a lift or completing extra reps are great examples of milestones to celebrate. Celebrate your workout streaks - how many days in a row you've committed and followed through. Treat yourself to something special, like a massage, make a toast on a healthy beverage with a workout buddy, or just revel in your hard work—your body (and mood) will thank you.

To build consistency, celebrate some of your wins—but not all. Neuroscientist Dr. Andrew Huberman calls this "Random Intermittent Reward Timing" (RIRT).[118] The idea is simple: unpredictable rewards spark more motivation than predictable ones. That's because irregular reinforcement activates the brain's dopamine system more powerfully, creating a sense of anticipation and making the behavior more likely to stick.

MOVEMENT AND INCREASED ENERGY

If you're not yet incorporating movement into your routine, it may seem difficult, especially if you're already struggling, and I want to level with you. The good news, if you're not feeling motivated, is that moving your limbs and core muscles will actually increase your energy levels. This is because exercise stimulates the release of adrenaline (epinephrine), which activates receptors on the vagus nerve—your gut-brain highway.[119] This activation enhances communication between the body and brain, leading to increased alertness and improved cognitive function.

ENJOY THE PROCESS

With the right mindset and strategies, you can create sustainable and even enjoyable habits. If you're intimidated by the idea of upping your level of movement, I hear you loud and clear. I've gone through periods of loathing exercise, especially because of my childhood injury-related chronic pain and difficult depressive symptoms over the years. However, I've learned to move strategically for mental health, and believe it or not, I've come to love several forms of exercise. We humans are incredibly adaptable. Not only can we get used to new habits, but we can also learn to enjoy things that at first seem hard.

Exercise doesn't have to feel like a chore. If you had mindset that exercise was difficult in the past, allow yourself to be open to the idea that a new movement routine can become enjoyable over time and with consistency. With some experimenting and patience, you can transform movement into something you look forward to—an act of self-care that energizes and uplifts you. Let's get going!

CHAPTER 10 SUMMARY

KEY CONCEPTS

1. **Movement can be as effective as antidepressants for some people.** Research shows that exercise can be just as effective as medication in alleviating depression and anxiety, but unlike pills, it requires consistent effort and engagement.

2. **The right type of movement matters.** Different types of exercise, from strength training to yoga and cardio, offer specific mental health benefits, and finding an enjoyable, sustainable routine is key to long-term success.

3. **Build a movement habit for mental well-being.** Using strategies like starting small, finding accountability, tracking progress, and pairing movement with joy can help turn exercise into a powerful tool for improving mood, energy, and resilience.

QUESTIONS:

1. **What types of movement could bring more joy into your life?** Reflect on the ideas from this chapter—are there any that feel exciting, uplifting, or motivating to add to your routine?

2. **What would help you feel more supported and energized around movement?** Think about the mindset shifts that resonated with you—what felt doable or inspiring, and how might those ideas help you take your next step?

3. **How can you celebrate your progress—big or seemingly small—each week or month?** Whether it's showing up, trying something new, or simply honoring your effort, what feels like a meaningful way to acknowledge your growth?

PART 3

PURPOSE

CHAPTER II

PURPOSE-DRIVEN PEACE

"Those who have a 'why' to live, can bear with almost any 'how'."

—Dr. Viktor E. Frankl,
Man's Search for Meaning

In the spring of 2017, my fourth child was born. At age 36, this pregnancy was by far the most challenging. A high-risk pregnancy diagnosis had me in and out of the hospital, taking prescription steroids, and then gestational diabetes medications. When our premature baby arrived, I was overjoyed—but the medical complications, sleepless nights, emergency birth, and the demands of caring for a newborn left me utterly depleted in terms of health, including, of course, my mental health.

Depression crept in almost immediately after our son's birth. My moods were fragile, compounded by hormonal shifts and the physiological fallout of a difficult pregnancy. I felt deeply committed to recovering, not just for my newborn, but for my family of six. However, by now, I knew that for me, pharmaceuticals alone wouldn't be the magic remedy. I began searching for alternative solutions.

Among the many doctors and healers I met, a few stand out as a pivotal turning point in my journey including Dr. Shiller, a functional MD who taught me about the power of an unexpected factor over the course of our first meeting. This *one factor* became a transformative remedy for me, and I've come to believe that it can be just as transformative for anyone.

A NEW PARADIGM FOR HEALING

By the time I saw Dr. Shiller in the fall of 2018, I was struggling with deep depression, chronic pain, and the physical toll of carrying an extra 30 unwanted pounds of inflammation and whatever else. Walking up and down the stairs in my home required gripping the railings to ease the pain from arthritis in my foot. I was in a rough moment, to say the least.

Dr. Shiller welcomed me into his office calmly and compassionately, gently holding a large glass mug of what appeared to be mushroom tea. His demeanor immediately put me at ease, making me feel seen, not as a collection of symptoms, but as a whole person. Instead of rushing to label me or scribble out a prescription, he listened intently as I summarized my struggles in the context of my life story. After listening intently, he shared an idea that forever shifted my perspective. Here is what he shared with me:

"There's a profound disconnect between what we can measure on an X-ray or MRI and a person's actual experience of health and well-being. For decades, studies have consistently shown that imaging findings—like disc bulges, arthritis, or joint degeneration—often don't correlate with pain or disability. The difference often lies not in the visible pathology, but in factors we can't measure on a scan—things like mindset, purpose, resilience, and the will to heal.

I was hooked listening to him, on the edge of my seat as he continued, *"I've seen patients with nearly identical injuries walk radically different paths. One might spiral into chronic pain, while another defies all odds and regains independence. **The key variable is often psychological and spiritual: a person's openness to growth, their belief in the possibility of healing, and their willingness to engage in the practices—whether physical, emotional, or spiritual—that move them forward.***

"True healing involves more than treating the body. It's about nurturing the whole person—body, mind, and spirit—and recognizing the incredible, often untapped, power we each hold to move toward vitality and wholeness."

A PRESCRIPTION FOR PURPOSE

Dr. Shiller paused—perhaps unaware of just how profoundly his words had landed—and then asked a question that opened the gate to an entirely new frontier in my healing journey. **What gives you a sense of purpose, Azi?**

Now, this was certainly a welcomed departure from my regular visits to the doctor. I immediately told him about my family—my husband and our four children—and how much meaning I found in my present opportunity to be a stay-at-home parent. **He listened, then gently asked, "And what about the parts of you outside of that role? What else matters to you?"**

The question stopped me in my tracks, and right away, I had a realization. Somewhere deep down, there was a creative spark within me—an inner drive to express myself more broadly. At that time, I had quietly started writing my first book, a collection of my favorite reflections on spirituality. I admitted to Dr. Shiller that I wasn't planning to share it publicly. I had convinced myself that keeping it private was an act of humility. He must have sensed that there was more to this story. He questioned my choice to keep my writing to myself, guiding me to gain insight that ultimately, I wasn't sharing my writing because I feared criticism and exposure. With time, I realized that sharing my work would be the generous choice, and a challenging exercise in emotional vulnerability.

HOW FEAR OF CRITICISM CAN BLOCK YOUR TRUE CALLING

Creating anything—whether it's a book, a speech, an original idea, or even a recipe—is an act of vulnerability. Putting yourself out there requires courage. It means risking criticism, rejection, or "failure." But it also means offering something of yourself to the world—something that might brighten someone's day or spark a shift, however seemingly small or grand.

If your work was critiqued when you were growing up, or if you went to schools where even your artwork was graded, you might have internalized the message that *creativity is risky*. Those critical adult voices can become part of your inner narrative without you even realizing it.

But here's the truth: showing up authentically—speaking your mind, sharing your feelings, putting your creations into the world—requires radical honesty. It means acknowledging what lights you up, and what fears could be holding you back. **Moving through that fear is often the very first step to living your purpose.**

FILLING THE PRESCRIPTION FOR PURPOSE

After receiving my 'prescription' for purpose that day, I began sharing excerpts of my book in small, manageable steps. First, it was just a post or two in a private Facebook group made up of trusted friends. As I started to see how the words resonated and felt increasingly safe expressing them, I gained the confidence to take the next step: publishing the book.

What worked about this approach was the pacing. I didn't rush. I took reasonable risks, one stage at a time. Each small act of sharing reminded me that it was safe to express myself. **If you're on a similar journey, know that you don't have to leap into the spotlight.** Invite a few trusted people into your creative process. Bounce ideas around. Let it be safe enough. Because while we'll never please everyone, we *can* share from an authentic place—and trust that the right people will connect with it.

And here's something else worth remembering: stepping into purpose doesn't have to mean writing a book, starting a podcast, or becoming a professional creative. For some people, it might simply mean doing *more* of what lights you up—taking that dance class, growing a garden, or volunteering in a way that brings you joy. For others, it's realizing the immense amount of purpose you're already fulfilling, even if you don't always see it that way.

Here's a great story to illustrate the point. In 1962, during a visit to the NASA Space Center, President John F. Kennedy reportedly stopped to speak with a janitor he saw carrying a broom. Curious, he introduced himself and asked the man what he was doing. Without hesitation, the janitor replied, "I'm helping put a man on the moon." That man's response can be a guiding light for all of us. It's a powerful reminder that purpose is for everyone. It's about how we *perceive* what we're doing—and recognizing the unique value in our contribution. That janitor understood he was part of something far greater than himself, and that belief infused his work with meaning.

There's another story that echoes this same idea. A traveler came across three bricklayers hard at work and asked each one what they were doing.

The first replied, "I'm laying bricks."

The second replied, "I'm building a wall."

The third smiled widely and replied, "I'm building a temple."

SAME TASK. COMPLETELY DIFFERENT MINDSET.

Whether we're writing books, raising children, volunteering, or showing up at our day jobs—it's the *meaning we attach* to what we're doing that shapes our sense of purpose. Living your purpose doesn't always mean starting something new. It means looking at what you're already doing through a different lens and realizing: *this matters*.

CHOOSING PURPOSE OVER EGO

There is a powerful spiritual idea that a state of enlightenment is one in which we do not allow ourselves to be offended. It's an idea I first heard from my friend Moshe Gersht, a wise and humble spiritual teacher. A simple way of understanding this is that **shame is the opposite of enlightenment**. Allowing ourselves to observe other people's reactions without personalizing them is a way to transcend our ego.

To make this tangible, you can remember: some people love puppies... and other people don't. It's a memorable reminder that no matter how pure, joyful, or well-intentioned something is, not everyone's going to like it. And that's okay. The opinions of other people only define you if you let them.

If you feel called to put something into the world—an idea, a message, a creative project, or even just to explore a new hobby—there's a reason for that. That inner nudge is no accident. Someone out there needs what you have to offer.

Whether or not everyone on the planet applauds you, what matters is that some people, yourself included, can benefit in ways that matter. **Your job in all of this is to keep showing up, creating, and leaning into a life of purpose—so you have a reason to get out of bed in the morning.** So that you can reconnect with the vitality, energy, and creativity that was divinely planted in *you*, and only you. This is how we reclaim our aliveness.

Think about it for a moment: You want to write that book, paint that painting, or speak from your heart. Chances are, you're being called to do this to serve the world. To innovate a product so that people can benefit, to make the world more colorful and beautiful, or to speak from the heart to promote truth and connection. It feels incredible to create and share because you are GIVING generously.

THE SPIRITUAL GIFT OF GIVING

In ancient Hebrew, the word for "give" is NATAN. Natan is a palindrome, spelled the same way forwards and backwards: NUN-TAV-NUN. We can understand this intentional spelling in one of two ways: what we give always comes back to us. Not necessarily from other people, as we can't control or expect this. However, the act and the joy of giving to the world is a way in which we also give to ourselves.

Finishing my first book in 2019 changed me. I shifted from being a passive *consumer* to an active *creator*. Since then, I've launched a podcast that's now top-ranked, helped start various initiatives, co-produced events, and built meaningful relationships along the way. Doors opened that I never could have imagined, and it all happened because I was willing to take a **reasonable risk.**

Part of transcending the ego is making peace with your creation, getting clear on your personal intention to put this into the world, and letting go of attachments to whatever feedback comes your way. As a child, I often threw away my own art projects if they weren't "perfect." Reframing failure as feedback hasn't come naturally—it's taken time and intention. But I've learned that both compliments and criticism can offer valuable insight into how your work is landing. If your creations are part of a growing business, this kind of feedback isn't just healthy—it's essential. The most important piece is to **stay clear on your intentions, enjoy the process of creating and giving, and let go of the idea that your value as a human being is at all tied to what other people think.**

STEPPING INTO YOUR PURPOSE

If you're afraid to start creating or expressing your PURPOSE more fully in the world, but you know deep down that you are being called to do so, you can begin by taking small steps. Share your ideas with a trusted circle before going public. Build your confidence slowly. The more you create, the less fear you'll feel, and the more you'll discover the fulfillment that comes from living with purpose. This is also like riding a bicycle; it may feel wobbly in the beginning, but once you get up and running, the wheels will gain momentum and you'll be flying high, enjoying the ride.

As I learned in that surprising first functional medicine session, our gifts are not meant to stay hidden. When you step into your purpose, you light up the world—and you'll find that it lights you up in return.

CHAPTER 11 SUMMARY

KEY CONCEPTS

1. **Purpose is a healing force.** A strong sense of purpose can be a powerful driver of resilience and well-being, helpful for overcoming physical and emotional challenges.

2. **Overcome fear and embrace creativity.** The journey to finding purpose often requires overcoming self-doubt and fear of criticism, as creating and sharing your work is an act of vulnerability that can also lead to personal growth and fulfillment.

3. **Giving is a path to meaning.** True purpose is rooted in contributing to others, and by stepping into your unique calling—whether through creating, innovating, or reframing your perspective around anything you're doing—you not only enrich the world but also experience a deep sense of joy.

QUESTIONS

1. **If you knew your idea would be a total success—loved, celebrated, and impactful—what would you create, say, or do?**

2. **Who might benefit from what you feel called to share or create?** How do you imagine it could unfold? What ripple effects might begin the moment you take that first step?

3. Is there something you might be avoiding by holding back your creativity? What fear or discomfort could be hiding underneath the resistance?

4. When you think about the kind of mark you want to leave on the world, what comes to mind? What kind of impact do you truly want to have?

5. Is there a way to reframe your mindset about the work your're doing to be more aligned with the 3rd response, "I'm building a temple," in the story of the three bricklayers?

PART 4

PEOPLE

POWER OF SOCIAL CONNECTION

*"Two are better than one... for if they
fall, one will lift up his friend."*

—Ecclesiastes, 4:9-10

The most powerful lesson I've ever learned about friendship didn't come during a personal crisis. It came when my dear friend Lisa—my soul sister of nearly thirty years—was living through one of the darkest moments of her life; one of the most devastating moments that any human can imagine.

On April 7, 2021, I opened Facebook for a routine check-in and saw a post that stopped me in my tracks. It was from Lisa, and it read:

"911: PRAY FOR NOAH WITH ALL YOUR MIGHT"

I knew that Lisa's 15-year-old son, Noah, had been struggling with severe health complications since being hit by a car a year earlier. I knew they'd seen doctor after doctor. But this—this was different. I felt it deep in my gut.

From across the world in Israel, all I could do at that moment was pray. I sent Lisa a message to let her know I was with her in spirit, desperate to offer something more.

Later that day, Lisa replied:

"Noah is gone. I can't anything."

I collapsed to my knees, sobbing in disbelief. Noah—the blonde-haired baby we held at his brit milah—the adorable toddler who lit up every room with his contagious, vibrant energy. He was the wise, creative, deeply sensitive soul who learned to rap brilliantly to express emotions too big for his young body.

Now, he was gone.

And in that moment of heartbreak, another instinct kicked in: *get there*.

Within minutes, my husband booked me a plane ticket, packed my bag, and drove me to the airport. Just 24 hours later, I arrived in Los Angeles in time for the funeral. On our way, another friend and I rushed to print photos of Noah. We needed to honor him, even in the smallest ways.

At the funeral, I sat in awe as Lisa and her husband Scott spoke with unimaginable strength, with their two beautiful children by their sides. Friends and educators described Noah as a shooting star—radiant, unforgettable, and gone too soon. His impact, they shared, would outlive his years.

The life-altering lesson in friendship came in the days that followed Noah's funeral.

According to Jewish tradition, the seven days after burial are for *shiva*—a time when the community visits the grieving family to offer comfort. Wanting to be helpful, I defaulted to doing—cleaning, tidying, making sure everything in the family home was in order. I thought I was doing everything right, since so many people would be coming through the home that week.

In truth, I had no clue what I was doing. I had never witnessed anything like this before in my life.

Fortunately, on Saturday night, Lisa called to offer some direction for the remaining days of shivah.

Her voice was gentle, loving, and also serious.

"I appreciate everything you're doing," she said. "But what I need most right now isn't help around the house. What's actually helping me most is when people just *sit* with me. When they *feel* this with me."

I felt a wave of shame at my own ignorance—and at the same time, a deep clarity. What mattered most in that moment wasn't dwelling on my misstep. It would be honoring what my friend truly needed: to show up and be as fully present as I possibly could.

This was the moment—the big lesson about true friendship I'll carry with me forever:

True friendship isn't always about *doing*. Yes, we're here to show up for each other—to celebrate life's beautiful moments and offer acts of kindness when someone's in need. All of this matters. But often, the most powerful gift we can offer isn't in *doing*, but instead it's in *being*.

Being present... and being willing to feel emotions alongside our friends.

Being a steady witness to someone else's grief—without trying to fix anything, or rushing to fill the silence.

This kind of friendship is sacred.

It's healing.

And it changes us—forever.

That experience with Lisa opened my heart. It revealed a depth of friendship I hadn't fully understood before, and it showed me what it means to truly show up for the people we care about.

FRIENDSHIP IS SACRED

Friendship has become a subject I've come to reflect on and value immensely. Part of this came from life experiences: moving multiple times—including a major move across the world in 2015—which meant starting over and building new relationships from scratch. And then, of course, when my mental health has had its downturns, friendships became central to my healing journey. I began to see **friendship not just as some sort of bonus in life, but as a non-negotiable; something vital and even sacred.**

From many, the loneliness and isolation during the pandemic clarified the vital importance of friendship. This shift has even led to some new approaches in the therapy world. Where therapy was once something people kept quiet about—especially in the '90s—today, it's become far more open. Not only are people talking about their experiences in therapy with friends, but some are even going *to therapy* with their friends.

There's a growing recognition that friendship is crucial to our mental, emotional, and even physical well-being. In fact, a new type of therapy has emerged in recent years that reflects just how much things have changed. While therapy used to be something whispered about—if it was mentioned at all—today, it's not uncommon for close friends to talk about therapy and even to go *together*.

Aminatou Sow and Ann Friedman, two longtime friends, even wrote a book on this concept: *Big Friendship: How We Keep Each Other Close*. Their relationship has been a meaningful, transformative force in both of their lives, but like all close relationships, it's had its challenges. Rather than let it fall apart, they chose to attend "friendship therapy" to strengthen their bond.

At one counseling center in Houston, Texas, therapist Barbie Atkinson uses friendship therapy in about one-fourth of her sessions.[120] What happens in these sessions is like what goes on for spouses; spending time understanding their unique attachment styles, communication methods, and the goals for their friendship. While I'm not evangelizing or promoting friendship therapy by any means, especially because for many people today, the cost of therapy can be prohibitive, I want to point out that **there's a great reason to place a high value on our friendships, especially our close ones. Whether you consider yourself an introvert, extrovert, or ambivert, the power of social connection for our mental and overall health is immense.**

Humans are wired for connection. Social relationships are not just a pleasant bonus in life—they are fundamental to our mental and physical well-being. Research consistently shows that people with strong social ties are healthier, happier, and live longer. On the other hand, loneliness and social isolation have been linked to depression, anxiety, and even premature death. Consider this 2023 advisory from the U.S. Surgeon General, equating the associated risks of loneliness and isolation to smoking 15 cigarettes daily.[121] The report emphasizes that a lack of social connection increases the risk of premature death by over 50%, underscoring the vital power of social connection. The advisory also calls for a National Strategy to Advance Social Connection, aiming to rebuild community social infrastructure.

This being said, if you're reading these statistics and starting to worry, wondering whether your friendships are "good enough" or what this means for your future, I want to pause here and remind you: *You are not a statistic.* Research reflects trends, definitely not destiny. The bell curve doesn't have to define your path. We're not here to aim for perfection—we're here for progress, self-love, and faith over fear. **If friendship is an area you're still growing in, that's okay. Friendship is the work of our lives.** This chapter is about hope, healing, and building the kinds of connections that will enhance our lives and our world, one day at a time, moving forward.

TECHNOLOGY AND RELATIONSHIPS

At this moment in history, we are living through a severe mental health crisis in *many* places around the globe. It's interesting because on one hand, human life has never been more convenient with the technological advancements that have made our day-to-day living less physically laborious. Modern life has afforded us with so many gifts, ways of saving time, and indispensable cures for what were once considered incurable diseases. **And yet, when it comes to mental health and so many other chronic diseases, we are witnessing a dramatic increase in suffering, loneliness, and even a widespread acceptance that half of modern society is simply "disordered."**

If we're more connected than ever, why is social isolation such a common experience? Adults, teens, and now even children are being diagnosed with mental health disorders without a clear scientific consensus as to why this is happening or what we can do about it. Suffering from mental health symptoms is rampant, and the well-being of our collective is at risk like never before unless we get to the bottom of this problem and, for the sake of humanity, join hands to solve it together.

CLOSE FRIENDSHIPS

Research affirms something many of us feel deep within: our close relationships in life matter immensely. Harvard's historic 85-year study on adult development—the most comprehensive of its kind—found that **the *quality* of our closest relationships has a greater impact on our happiness and longevity than wealth, status, or external success.**[122] The big takeaway from their nearly a century of research is clear: it's not about how *many* friends you have or how *much* money you make—**it's the people you walk closely with through life who shape your well-being in the most meaningful ways.**

SOCIAL CONTAGION

What fascinates me about relationships—especially the close kind—is how much we can shape each other. The phrases, words, and underlying tones we pick up from those closest to us often become part of our own inner dialogue. Over time, their energy and presence begin to" live" inside of us in a certain way.

There's a popular saying in the personal development world: *"You become the sum of the five people you spend the most time with,"* and science backs this up. In the 1970s, sociolinguist Howard Giles developed what's known as Communication Accommodation Theory (CAT), which explains how **we naturally start to mirror the people we're around**—matching their pace, tone, accents, and even word choices, often without realizing it.[123] This kind of subtle syncing is especially common among close friends, and it deepens connection and mutual understanding.

Even more recently, researchers found that people who use similar language patterns—whether in student essays or Amazon reviews—are more likely to become friends.[124] This is a reminder that friendship doesn't just shape how we feel—it can shape who we become.

So the deeper question to consider is: Who are you choosing to walk with in life? And how are those relationships shaping the way you speak, think, and grow?

CREATING CONNECTION INTENTIONALLY

What's also interesting is that when you repeat someone's words or slightly mimic their gestures, this fosters a sense of connection and understanding between people. It creates rapport and strengthens our interpersonal bonds. This technique is called "mirroring," and is so powerful that experts in critical hostage negotiation settings use it. Former FBI hostage negotiator Chris Voss explains that mirroring "gets (the other side) talking and creates the opportunity for them actually to present you with *your* deal, only they thought it was their idea."[125] This is one of the quickest ways, when done with intention, to create a feeling of connection with another person.

THE PURPOSE OF FRIENDSHIP

What *should* our intentions be when it comes to making and sustaining close friendships, and *how* do we create those close social connections? For life's biggest questions, such as these, I often turn to the ancient wisdom that has endured for thousands of years.

There's a beautiful idea in Ancient Jewish spiritual wisdom explaining that **the purpose of friendship is to help us evolve spiritually.** So much importance is placed on this that the famed Ethics of Our Fathers instructs, **"acquire for yourself a friend."**[126] The original word used in Hebrew, translated as "acquire," and pronounced "*leek-note,*" also translates to "buy."

SPIRITUAL GROWTH

The commentators explain the deeper meaning: a friend is, ideally, someone who can help you grow in the most valuable ways. Now, if you don't identify as a spiritual person, I want to explain how it's also a *practical* idea. Growing spiritually in this context is to grow *ethically* and to maximize your human potential: doing the right thing, looking after your health, being a responsible citizen, pursuing justice, functioning at your best, and performing acts of kindness are a few examples. So, the idea here is to seek out friends who will bring you up and support you in growing into the most fully expressed version of your authentic self.

Friendship, also according to ancient wisdom, is not about *sameness.* It's about bringing positive influences into your life, which will, in turn, bring out the best in you. If you seek out a friend who values fitness, chances are that you'll become more active through the friendship. I'm willing to bet that you've also got positive qualities, even unique to your friend's, that can elevate your friend, too. Friendship is an opportunity to share your unique qualities and help bring out the one-of-a-kindness in everyone you meet.

Beyond the spiritual 'transaction' going on, close friendship brings people a sense of psychological safety. Over the past twenty-five years or so, I've made some phenomenal friends, and honestly, many more than I ever imagined possible. But, truth be told, in the first two decades of my life, I had a really bad habit of sabotaging friendships.

While I didn't understand *why* I was doing it at the time, looking back, I understand that I was subconsciously self-protecting, which turns out to be a common reason people sabotage their relationships. This can look like repeatedly breaking commitments, pushing people away, or even picking fights and arguments for no apparent reason. It can also look like avoidance, jealousy, defensiveness, criticism, or trust difficulties.

THE SCIENCE OF RELATIONSHIPS

To understand the science of building relationships, we can begin by examining what destroys them. According to the data, twelve specific behaviors are attributed to sabotaging relationships. One tool, the **Relationship Sabotage Scale (RSS),** consists of 12 items designed to measure self-sabotaging behaviors in romantic relationships.[127] While the RSS has been researched in the context of couples, it can also give you a sense of your tendencies in close friendships. If you're curious about a possible tendency to sabotage, you can use this self-assessment tool based on the RSS. For each statement, rate how much it applies to you on a scale of 1 (**Strongly Disagree**) to 5 (**Strongly Agree**):

Relationship Sabotage Scale (RSS) Items:

1. I avoid being vulnerable in my relationships.
2. I find it difficult to trust my partner.
3. I frequently expect my relationships to fail.
4. I have trouble communicating my needs effectively.
5. I tend to push my partner away when I feel close to them.
6. I assume the worst about my partner's intentions.
7. I find it challenging to resolve conflicts in a healthy way.
8. I feel insecure about my partner's commitment to me.
9. I am quick to become defensive during arguments.
10. I struggle to maintain emotional closeness with my partner.
11. I tend to dwell on potential relationship problems instead of enjoying the present.
12. I have difficulty setting or respecting boundaries in my relationships.

Scoring: Add up your scores for all 12 items.

- **Low (12–24):** Minimal sabotaging tendencies.

- **Moderate (25–39):** Some sabotaging behaviors may affect your relationships; consider areas for improvement.

- **High (40–60):** Significant sabotaging tendencies; these behaviors may be interfering with your relationship satisfaction.

Your score can guide you to reflect on potential patterns in your relationships and give you a sense of what you can work on. The main behaviors you're uncovering by taking this test point to potential levels of **defensiveness, trust difficulty, and lack of relationship skills.**

Please remember, no matter what your score was on this assessment, it can change! If you've been sabotaging your relationships, you can't criticize or shame yourself out of it. The past is in the past, and every action moving forward paves the way to the future you desire.

The most effective way of growing our capacities sustainably is through compassion with ourselves. This is because most sabotaging behaviors are done for the purpose of self-protection, such as shielding ourselves from future rejections. As human beings, we are wired to survive, and this means doing whatever we can to stay safe.

PLAYING IT SAFE

Human beings are wired to seek both physical and psychological safety. Evolutionary psychology explains that we are biologically wired to protect ourselves from harm—a survival mechanism that was essential in primitive times. Early humans faced constant threats from predators, harsh environments, and scarce resources. It is believed that because of this, **the human brain has evolved to prioritize safety, developing a heightened sensitivity to potential danger.**[128] This "fight, flight, or freeze" response, governed by the amygdala, allowed early humans to react quickly to threats and increased their chances of survival.[129] While this protective mechanism was highly adaptive in primitive environments, it can be *maladaptive* today.

The same instincts that once shielded humans from physical danger can get in the way of your ability to be emotionally vulnerable and build deep connections. For instance, avoiding perceived "threats" like rejection or criticism may lead to withdrawal, self-isolation, or an inability to communicate openly. **While rooted in an adaptive instinct to play it safe, these fear-based responses can discourage us from speaking from the heart, expressing our emotions, or doing anything remotely vulnerable — key components of emotional growth and intimacy.** As a result, what once kept us alive can limit our ability to thrive in today's social and emotional contexts.

By recognizing these deeply ingrained and universal dynamics, it's possible to unlearn behaviors and replace them with healthier ones. Again, the key to growth here is being compassionate with yourself in the process.

THE POWER OF CLOSE RELATIONSHIPS

Close relationships can have tremendous mental and overall health benefits. [130] They reduce feelings of loneliness, provide emotional and practical support, and mitigate stress. **People with stronger social ties have lower blood pressure, reduced cortisol, and stronger immune systems.** Social interactions stimulate the brain, improving cognitive function and reducing the risk of dementia.

It's important to remember that the research around relationships and health points to **close relationships** as the hallmark of our well-being. Specifically, these types of relationships have three things in common:

1. **Emotional Intimacy:** A deep sense of mutual understanding and trust.

2. **Reliability:** Confidence that one can depend on the other in times of need.

3. **Low Conflict Levels:** Relationships characterized by minimal conflict and high levels of warmth.

If you're considering shifting or expanding your close social circle, keeping these three pillars of close friendship in mind is a great idea. Seek out people who, as much as possible, understand themselves and their emotions and have the capacity for the emotional intimacy you're seeking. The opposite of the sabotaging behaviors are the actions that build friendship:

- Practicing grounded vulnerability in relationships.
- Offering trust, consciously and over time.
- Having a hopeful, optimistic, and growth mindset.
- Creating space for meaningful connection.
- Believing in others' good intentions.
- Prioritizing peace over conflict.

- Being rooted with a strong sense of self-worth.
- Receiving feedback with openness and not defensiveness.
- Allowing emotional closeness and connection.
- Choosing faith over fear, and not spiraling into overthinking.
- Honoring your limits with compassionate boundaries.

If you're rattling off this list and thinking what I'm thinking, then we can probably agree: it's unlikely or impossible to find a human being on planet earth that does not struggle with any of these twelve tendencies, even if to a small degree. Relationships are the *work of our lives,* and they have the power to inspire our growth. With all of this in mind, we can focus inward on embodying the characteristics needed to foster meaningful and close relationships. We can learn to let go of our shortcomings and practice giving the benefit of the doubt when other people in our lives are doing their best in ways we cannot fully understand, including ourselves.

BEFRIENDING OURSELVES

Building close relationships begins with befriending ourselves. Understanding our human tendencies, aiming to do our best, and having compassion on ourselves in the process is a great start. Invest time and energy into understanding the goals and expectations of the people who matter most to you first. Take an inventory of your calendar and the time you spend socializing, and make sure you're investing your time consciously into the relationships you want to foster. With the health benefits of maintaining close relationships in mind, you can understand why this investment is so worthwhile.

From the bottom of my heart, I want you to know that one of the most liberating parts of my healing journey has been learning to forgive myself for my past missteps.

Through deep inner work and also in the safety of structured therapy, I came to see how certain experiences from my childhood had been quietly haunting me—so deeply, in fact, that I had blocked some of them from memory for years. Decisions I made as a young teenager—impulsive, misguided, and shaped by survival—were still echoing subconsciously inside me years later.

But something shifted when I finally found the courage to bring those memories into the light, to speak them aloud in a space of compassion and safety. I could see, with absolute clarity, that I was doing the best I knew how to do at the time. And even more freeing—I realized I'm no longer that same person.

Processing the past doesn't mean reliving it—it means releasing it. And when done safely, it can both set you free and set you up to become your own biggest advocate.

Our social connections are a cornerstone of our mental health and overall well-being. While modern life often leaves little time for cultivating relationships, nurturing these bonds is one of the best investments you can make. Starting now, you can create a thriving social environment that supports your mental health and overall well-being for years to come.

Using the ECHO method to enrich your social connections:

1. **Education:** Learn about the importance of connection and the risks of isolation. Learn about yourself, your patterns, and tendencies. Learn about building meaningful relationships. Consider: Who will most likely support you in evolving into the best version of yourself? Who sees the good in you? How can you shift your focus to see more of the good in others?

2. **Curiosity:** Get curious about how cultivating and maintaining a few close friendships could evolve your well-being. How could prioritizing close friendships affect your confidence, self-compassion, or sense of purpose? How could fostering close friendships lead to lifestyle changes?

3. **Healing:** Implement one intentional step in the coming weeks, like getting together with a friend or even catching up over the phone. If you're starting from scratch, this could look like joining a local meetup group based on one of your interests, or visiting a local community center.

4. **Observation:** Notice how these efforts impact your mood, stress levels, and overall sense of well-being. Notice what parts of your interactions felt supportive, positive, and memorable. Make a conscious decision to implement the upgrades that support your thriving.

Your social connectedness begins with your cultivating an intention, befriending yourself, and then befriending another. Here's to the everlasting power of friendship enriching our world.

CHAPTER 12 SUMMARY

KEY CONCEPTS

1. **Understand the importance of friendship.** In contrast to past stigma around therapy, a new trend sees friends attending therapy together to strengthen their relationships, recognizing the crucial role friendships play in mental and overall well-being.

2. **The science of social connection is real.** Research shows that strong social bonds improve happiness, longevity, and health, while loneliness poses serious risks, emphasizing the need for intentional efforts to cultivate close, supportive relationships.

3. **Build meaningful friendships for growth and well-being.** True friendships are built on emotional intimacy, reliability, and low conflict, with ancient wisdom and modern psychology alike highlighting their role in personal development, self-improvement, and overall life satisfaction.

QUESTIONS

1. Who do you want to be emulating most, and how can you spend more time around these people?

2. Who is most likely to help you grow into the best version of yourself? Who sees the good in you?

3. What personality traits or relationship patterns have you been drawn to in the past? What kind of close friendships do you want to cultivate in the future?

SPIRITUALITY

"Miracles are all around us."

—Ruchoma Shain

As a teen, one of my safe havens was the bookstore. With a latte in one hand and a book in the other, I'd spend weekends lost in teachings about spirituality and personal growth. At one point, I even took a part-time job at a local psychic bookstore so I could immerse myself in the metaphysical world as much as possible.

This early curiosity eventually led me to several institutes for spiritual learning in Jerusalem from 2003 to 2004.

One morning, I wandered into the quiet library in one of those spaces. As I scanned the four walls of bookshelves, my shoulder brushed against one of them, and a single book tumbled down and hit me on the head.[131] The cover was sky blue, scattered with wisps of clouds. The title read *All for the Best*, and I opened it, immediately drawn in.

Just then, a young woman burst into the room just as I got a few pages into this new book.[132] "There's an older woman nearby who just had surgery," she said. "She's alone and needs help."

"What's her name?" I asked. "Where does she live?"

"Ruchoma Shain. Two blocks south, number 70, apartment 8."

My eyes dropped down to the book in my hands. Ruchoma Shain was the author of this very book. What were the chances?

There are moments in life that seem to defy logic—where the timing is too exact, the unfolding too purposeful to dismiss as merely coincidence. This was one of them.

I raced out of the library and made my way to the address. Breathless, I stood in front of a heavy metal door. "Come right in," a soft voice called from inside.

The apartment was modest, its walls lined with books that glowed in the morning light. In front of the window sat a gentle-looking woman in an armchair. "Thank you for coming," she said. "My children will be here from New Jersey soon. Until then, could you kindly help me up?" I reached out, and she clasped my hands with surprising strength. We moved to the kitchen table, where a tea kettle sat warming on the stove.

"What brings you all the way here?" she asked.

I hadn't fully explained the purpose of this year-long trip to anyone—not even to myself. But her stillness invited honesty.

"I'm searching for something," I said. "I don't know what exactly... but I know there's more to life than what I can see or touch." She listened, eyes bright with interest. "Miracles," she said softly, "are all around us."

I paused, stunned. "You won't believe what happened to me this morning..."

She smiled knowingly, just as the kettle began to whistle. I poured us tea and returned to the table. "You see this phone?" she said, pointing to the beige landline on the table. "We think of it as *just* technology—but it's miraculous, really. We're connected to people across the world with the press of a few buttons."

"When we wake up and can see, hear, think, and breathe—this too is a miracle," she continued. **"And the more you recognize the miracles already in your life, the more you'll begin to see them everywhere."**

Her words landed deeply within me. My eyes welled with tears. Truth, I've learned, can be both simple and profound at the same time. This experience was an unexpected, unexplainable moment of quiet awakening. It marked the beginning of a journey—not just to learn something new, but to remember what she taught me: There's more to this life than we can perceive with our physical senses alone.

Guidance can come through seemingly simple moments—a book falling off a shelf, an unexpected encounter with a stranger, or any number of "ordinary" events that wind up making extraordinary impact. This moment became my own short course in miracles, teaching me that awareness of and gratitude for the miraculous can transform the way we experience everyday life, revealing more and more of the miraculous.

WHAT IS SPIRITUALITY, ANYWAY?

Spirituality is generally defined as a sense of connection to *something* greater than yourself, or the experience of interconnection with all of life. Sometimes people let go of believing in *something* greater after witnessing events in life that don't seem to make sense, like why bad things happen to good people and vice versa. Whether you consider yourself religious or spiritual, or neither, we can probably all agree about a few fundamental spiritual truths:

1. No one understands the origin of our existence completely, where the universe "ends," or exactly what happens after we die, and it's quite possible that no living human being ever will.

2. Human beings can be incredibly bright and capable, but the beyond-genius Force that has created this universe is beyond our human comprehension.

3. In order to live in a more just and harmonious world, there are basic interpersonal agreements, "team humanity" will need to make sure that people will, once and for all, have the rights and freedoms everyone deserves. Somehow, we need to agree on basic, fundamental rights for all human beings to achieve a state of harmony and coexistence.

4. Prioritizing profit over the basic fundamental rights and well-being of human beings is not spiritual and has disrupted the harmony of our planet and its inhabitants.

5. Oppressing, enslaving, or brutalizing people in the name of religion is not and will never be the answer to creating a world order.

6. Many of us have had moments that feel unexplainable—like déjà vu, meaningful coincidences, vivid dreams with answers, or chance encounters that feel guided. Whether you see these as spiritual or simply part of the mystery of life, they point us to a dimension of reality that's hard to explain but can be deeply experienced.

EYES OF SOUL

Taking a spiritual perspective and viewing the world with Eyes of Soul is a grateful acknowledgement of the awe and wonder of this universe. It can include reconnecting with nature, truly befriending yourself and others, and reveling in this uniquely human experience on planet Earth.

Eyes of Soul is a teaching from Rav Abraham Isaac Kook, one of the most influential Jewish mystics and philosophers of the 20th century. He introduced the idea of perceiving the world not only through our physical senses, but through what he called the *"eyes of the soul."*

This concept encourages us to move beyond surface-level appearances and tune into a deeper, more expansive way of seeing—**one that recognizes meaning, beauty, and interconnectedness even in the ordinary.** Whether you interpret this as spiritual intuition, heightened awareness, or simply a mindful way of engaging with life, the invitation is the same: **to be present enough to witness the extraordinary within the everyday.**

Rav Kook writes:

> "If you desire, human being, look at the light of God's Presence in everything. Look at the Eden of spiritual life and how it blazes into each corner and crevice of life, spiritual and of this world, right before your eyes of flesh and soul..."
> — Rav Kook, *Orot HaKodesh*[133]

Spirituality has always fascinated me, and a few other pivotal teachings have been particularly instrumental in guiding me to reclaim my mental health and thrive.

WHO IS WISE?

An ancient Jewish ethical tractate known as Ethics of our Fathers poses the question, "Who is wise?" We contemplated this question earlier when considering what kind of medical professionals to seek out, and it's relevant to fostering friendships, too. Before we proceed, take a moment to think about what wisdom means to you. Who, in your Eyes of Soul, is wise?

Ethics of our fathers provides a profound answer: The one who is wise is the "one who learns from all." This points to the wisdom in humility, and the spiritual truth that everyone you meet has something to teach you, as we explored in the chapter about the power of friendship. Through the Eyes of Soul, every single person you meet in life is here to teach you something and help you fulfill your life's mission.

OPPORTUNITIES TO GROW

Some people might act in ways that you might feel inspired to emulate, reminding you of something in yourself that you want to nurture. If your interaction with another person is bothersome, with a spiritual perspective, it can still be an opportunity for growth if you ask yourself: How can you maintain your values in this moment? What can you learn? The spiritual practice here is to realize that it's all a gift and an opportunity to learn.

Being in the presence of someone who bothers you for whatever reason can also be a powerful opportunity to get to know yourself better and to grow. When you observe someone doing something you don't instinctively or rationally like, try asking yourself, "how am I also like this?" or in other words, "what is this person reminding me about myself that I might be avoiding?"

The answer may not be a direct one-to-one comparison, but asking the question can open a powerful doorway to self-awareness and meaningful inner growth.

BENEFIT OF THE DOUBT

The next spiritual principle that can revolutionize your mental health is giving other people the benefit of the doubt. Giving someone the **benefit of the doubt** is also spoken about in Ethics of our Fathers, and it refers to assuming positive intent and seeking a favorable interpretation of another person's actions, even if their behavior is questionable. Giving someone the benefit of the doubt is absolutely not the same thing as allowing yourself to be taken advantage of. In general, giving someone the benefit of the doubt is drawing the conclusion that the other person has *good intentions* underneath an action that doesn't make complete sense to us. Taking on this perspective fosters compassion and frees you from walking around with the heavy burdens of resentment or anger on your shoulders.

Giving others the benefit of the doubt acknowledges that we rarely know the full story behind someone's choices. It's kind of like this: you're driving behind a car on the road that comes to a sudden halt. As much as you might want to honk at the car for driving recklessly, for all you know, there's much more going on: a pothole in the road, or a child crossing the road that you are simply unable to see. When people aren't behaving in ways that make sense to you, and when you can't see the full picture (which is basically always) and don't have proof to believe otherwise, always give someone the benefit of the doubt. In doing this, you'll be reducing your own stress and anxiety by shifting your nervous system out of fight-or-flight and into more relaxed states.

PRAYER

You don't have to be religious to find value in this concept—its essence may still resonate. Prayer is a powerful opportunity to connect with our highest intentions and align with our greatest potential. It is more than just asking for something; it is a way of attuning ourselves to a deeper truth, refining our desires, and clarifying how what we seek can contribute to the greater good. Across several ancient traditions, prayer has a structured format—beginning with praise, moving into a request, and concluding with gratitude. This structure frames prayers with humility and appreciation and reminds us that true connection with The Infinite is a two-way relationship.

If you don't identify as religious or spiritual, you can still benefit from the format of this practice: **setting clear intentions, aligning with your highest values, and opening yourself to possibilities beyond your immediate control.** We can all benefit by focusing on what truly matters, expressing gratitude, and recognizing that while you can take action toward your goals, some outcomes are beyond your influence. **Letting go of rigid expectations and trusting the process can bring peace and a deeper sense of connection to yourself and the world around you.**

A particularly powerful prayer practice that can bring about miracles involves getting crystal clear on your intentions: Why do you want what you're praying for? (This kind of "why" isn't about second-guessing your desire—it's an invitation to go deeper: What is this intention really for? What's the deeper purpose or hoped-for impact?) You can set aside time to gently and compassionately ask yourself "why," again and again, and listen deeply to every possible answer. This process ensures you that your requests are aligned with the greater good and recognizes how the fulfillment of your intention can bring about a more whole world.

What *needs* does your prayer fulfill? Whether you're praying for world peace or for a livelihood, be as specific as you can about why this outcome is so important to you, and why it will help you and/or others fulfill their full potential. In ancient Hebrew, the word for prayer is "Avodah," translating as both "work" and "prayer." Perhaps this is hinting to us that prayer is not about making a passive wish, but rather it's about an active partnership, where our role is to take aligned action toward manifesting our prayers.

TRUST AND ACCEPTANCE IN PRAYER

At its core, prayer is also about trust and acceptance. While we can pour our hearts into our prayers, having Eyes of Soul acknowledges that whatever comes to pass is ultimately for the good. This can be extremely hard in a difficult moment, asking ourselves, "Why me? Why did this have to happen to *me*?" Life can unfold in ways we don't expect or fully understand, but with one spiritual perspective shift, we can learn to see reality as it is—trusting that even in disappointment or challenge, there is a higher wisdom at play. This one spiritual shift is as follows: **Life is not happening *to* you, but rather, life is happening *for* you.**

On a psychological level, this mindset takes you out of a victim mentality, the powerless state where you have no control over your destiny. Asking, how is this *for* me, even in a difficult time, allows you to keep learning, searching for new opportunities, and expanding your life no matter what comes your way. Stories of resilience don't emerge from ease; they arise from adversity. Think about Nelson Mandela, who endured 27 years in prison and emerged to lead South Africa to reconciliation. And Dr. Viktor Frankl, who survived the Holocaust and transformed his suffering into *Man's Search for Meaning*, a guide to finding purpose even in hardship. And how about Malala Yousafzai, who at age 15 survived being shot by the Taliban for advocating girls' education, and then went on to become the youngest Nobel Prize laureate. Most recently, the words of Agam Berger, a 20-year-old young woman, who was held captive by the violent terrorist group Hamas in Gaza for 482 days. In her WSJ op-ed, she reminds us that spiritual freedom can endure even in the most harrowing conditions.[134] Her unwavering faith became a source of strength for her, proof that even when the body is confined, the spirit can remain profoundly free.

The strength these humans have shown is, to me, beyond comprehension. From whereever you are starting and with whatever you're facing, you can remember this:

Those who embrace life's challenges as opportunities for growth open the door to infinite possibility.

THE HUMAN INCLINATIONS

At the heart of many religions is the belief that human beings have both positive and negative inclinations, which influence their choices. In Judaism, there are two inclinations: one toward good and one toward evil. What does this mean, exactly, and how can we understand this in the context of our spiritual journey?

In 2020, I had the opportunity to interview Rabbi Dr. Abraham Twerski on this topic, and he shared the most insightful piece of wisdom on this topic I've ever heard.[135] Rabbi Dr. Twerski (1930–2021) was a renowned Hasidic rabbi, psychiatrist, and addiction specialist who integrated Jewish wisdom with modern psychology to help people overcome addictions and live their best lives. He authored over 90 books, founded the Gateway Rehabilitation Center, and was widely respected for his compassionate, insightful approach to healing, blending philosophical teachings with psychological expertise.

Rabbi Dr. Twerski explained in our interview that the *evil inclination* isn't actually our drive to sin or do "bad" things. As he explained, the evil inclination is actually the embodiment of a person's self-doubt. **In other words, the root of all human behavior that throws the spiritual balance of the universe out of order is…. people doubting themselves!!!**

There are endless applications of this idea. For starters, by believing in yourself, you can create and share things with the world: art, poems, businesses, ideas, speeches ... you name it. In all seriousness, this also means that when we look around the world and witness entire societies being swept into violent and hateful ideologies, at the root of their susceptibility to these harmful ideologies is their fragile self-image. *People who do not believe in themselves or their capacity for good can become extremely dangerous to themselves and to our society.*

During graduate school, I developed a strong interest in understanding the roots of deviant behavior—to move past pathologizing and uncover both what drives deviance and how transformation is possible. For my doctoral dissertation, I conducted research in some of Los Angeles's most economically and socially marginalized high schools. I also volunteered in the Los Angeles juvenile prison, where I encountered students who had once sat in classrooms just like those I was studying.

My focus was on understanding why some at-risk youth go on to defy the odds and build lives that are seen as successful and meaningful, while others, despite their strength and potential, struggle to break through. I wasn't just looking for a formula for success but rather trying to explore the deeper story: the conditions, relationships, and internal resources that can help a young person rise, even when the odds are stacked against them.

I discovered rather quickly why most of these young people struggle, both in the research, and on my first day driving into these neighborhoods, after speaking with community members. These young people face huge obstacles and ongoing traumas, even on a daily basis. By reviewing research and interviewing educators, I also discovered one defining factor that sets the successful few apart from the rest.

BELIEFS AND RELATIONSHIPS: THE KEYS TO TRANSFORMATION

Here's what I discovered through the research: Students who are able to overcome adversity and thrive against the odds have at least one key relationship with an adult who genuinely believes in them—someone who cares for their physical and emotional needs and holds them to high expectations. This one key relationship is, in most cases, the difference between success and failure. The problem, however, is that it's hard for teachers to do this for every student. With increasing class sizes, the pressure of standardized testing, and limited resources, especially in low-income area schools, it's very difficult for one teacher to be *the* key person in the lives of all of their students.

Reflecting back on your school experiences, were you one of the lucky students to have an adult guiding you through the process? Have you been blessed with role models in your life who believed in you? Have you received mentoring over the years to guide you in achieving your goals? Having someone in your life who you respect, who will believe in you, and who will mentor you is priceless. While we can all benefit from this, there are no guarantees that everyone will be blessed and lucky enough to have that one special teacher in school or, later on in life, a business mentor who helps them get to the next level.

BECOMING YOUR OWN GREATEST ADVOCATE

By internalizing the spiritual idea that **self-doubt is the root of all evil,** we can also conclude that **believing in ourselves is the root of all good.** This isn't about thinking you're *better* than anyone else—it's about recognizing that you are **perfectly unique,** with a role and mission in the world that no one else can fulfill.

Becoming your greatest advocate requires reaching deep within yourself, accessing the wisest, most loving, faithful part of your being, and allowing that part to flourish. It's about truly knowing yourself and seeing past the fear-based, self-protective, totally normal human behaviors that may have tricked you into believing that you're selfish (or disordered). At your core, **you are a pure soul of light, a piece of The Infinite, wanting nothing more than to illuminate the path for others.** By continuing to recognize the good you're doing and believe in your potential to grow and thrive, you can be one of the wise and loving teachers that you need the most, holding yourself to high standards and compassionately caring for yourself along the way. Becoming your own greatest supporter will help you advocate for yourself in all mental health related spaces, too, which will only benefit your well-being.

In a world that often profits from your self-doubt, one of the most radical things you can do to reclaim your mental health and truly thrive is to believe that you can.

CHAPTER 13 SUMMARY

KEY CONCEPTS

1. **View spirituality as connection and awe.** Spirituality is a deep sense of connection to all of life, an embracing of the mystery of existence, and an awareness of the awe-inspiring synchronicities that point to something beyond human understanding.

2. **Prioritize wisdom and compassion in relationships.** Spiritual wisdom involves learning from every person we encounter, giving others the benefit of the doubt, and having compassion, which can improve our overall health.

3. **Overcoming self-doubt is a spiritual matter.** The greatest spiritual battle is our battle with self-doubt, which can lead to destructive behaviors. Believing in oneself fosters creativity, resilience, and the ability to make your unique and indelible mark on the world like only you can.

QUESTIONS

1. Looking back on your school years, was there someone— an adult, a teacher, a mentor—who really saw you and guided you along the way? Have you had people in your life who believed in you when you needed it most? Who have been the voices of encouragement helping you move toward your goals?

2. Think of a recent moment when someone rubbed you the wrong way or triggered something in you. What might that interaction be reflecting back to you about your own inner work? Is there a way to reframe the experience through a lens of growth or spiritual insight?

3. In what areas of your life do you tend to doubt yourself the most? Take a moment to name them honestly. That clarity is the first step toward becoming your own strongest supporter—and learning to show up for yourself with compassion and courage.

SENSORY HEALING MODALITIES FOR MIND, BODY, AND SPIRIT

"Sometimes it's the simplest self-improvement practices that lead to the most dramatic transformations."

—Benjamin Farley,
Founder of Unchained Earth &
Creator of The Unwind Machine

At first glance, a chapter on sensory healing might not seem like the obvious place to reflect on my seven inpatient stays in psychiatric wards. But in truth, it's the perfect place, and I'll explain to you exactly why.

I've held off on sharing the details of my psychiatric 'hospitalizations,' in part because most of them resembled the worst of what people imagine and had zero therapeutic value: these were sterile, fluorescent-lit facilities that reeked of chemical-based cleaners. Places where human suffering is often met with coldness, confinement, and condescension.

These are places sealed off from the outside world, where I was stripped of my shoelaces, my dignity, and sometimes even my sense of humanity. I've shuffled down the halls, trembling with pharmaceutical-induced akathisia—one of the most distressing side effects of psych meds[136]—like a ghost, among others who were deeply dismissed, their pain often intensified by being treated more like violent criminals than patients.

I don't think it will be helpful for me to recount every detail of those experiences in these pages. But I would be remiss not to tell you about my final stay, in the summer of 2022, because something happened there that was different.

It took place in central Israel, not far from my home, in a publicly funded psychiatric hospital. It was far from a perfect situation, but what set it apart was the environment, and the way it gently reintroduced me to the healing power of the senses.

Instead of being locked indoors, we were invited to spend time outside. The grounds were humble but expansive, with towering, forest-like trees and a vibrant green lawn where we sat each afternoon—shoes off, sun on our skin—letting the healing power of nature and human connection sink deep into our souls. I connected with people from all walks of life, and what united us deeply was our shared humanity in this vulnerable chapter of our lives.

There was a small organic garden filled with color and life—we would walk over and pick purple grapes straight from the vine, tear fresh cabbage leaves from the earth, and eat them right there in the moment.

The program also brought in sensory healing practitioners. I experienced laughter therapy for the first time and laughed so hard I slid off my chair. I also tried dog therapy and felt an unexpected softening, a kind of safety and connection that animals uniquely provide. We broke ceramic tiles to express our inner shattering, then reassembled them into mosaics—raw, imperfect, and even beautiful. Something shifted for me during those days. **Sitting on the grass with my unlikely tribe of fellow patients—sunlight on our faces, grass beneath our toes—I remembered something buried beneath the diagnosis, the chaos, and the pain.**

I was still a human being, and I was intricately connected to nature.

Like nature, I began to feel permission to move through seasons, to shed old leaves—however painfully—with the quiet knowledge that in time, new ones would grow in their place, more expansive than what came before.

My renewal didn't come from one big breakthrough. It came through small, daily moments of reconnection to nature, fellow humans, and myself.

These moments inspired healing, showing me how senses can be powerful portals—pathways to calm, clarity, and a palpable sense of aliveness.

Each of us can improve our overall health and wellness through sensory protocols—simple, evidence-based practices that support nervous system regulation, reduce stress, and enhance mental clarity. These tools aren't at all exclusive to clinical settings; many can be implemented independently, starting today from the comfort of wherever life finds you.

In this chapter, you're invited to explore a buffet of these sensory protocols using the ECHO method—approaching each one with Education, Curiosity, Healing, and Observation. You're invited to try on what speaks to you and tune in to how you feel—mind, body, and spirit—before, during, and after each practice.

Some of what follows may feel familiar—protocols we've touched on in earlier chapters—but you'll also discover new and accessible tools to help you feel more grounded, more empowered, and more connected to yourself and the world around you. I'll also say in advance that there are an infinite number of sensory protocols. This list includes quite a few, compiled in place so that you can come back to them at any point and use what serves you at any moment. Let's begin.

EYES:

As it has been said, the eyes are the windows to the soul. This quote is often understood to mean that you can see someone's soul through their eyes. It's also interesting to consider that what you look at and engage with visually enters your mind, body, and soul, and can impact your overall sense of health and well-being.

LIGHT:

Remember that your body is intrinsically tied to nature. Looking at the positive mental health outcomes of several indigenous societies, we find a direct link between mental health and sleeping according to the sun's natural rhythm.

I. PRIORITIZE MORNING SUNLIGHT EXPOSURE.

When you wake up in the morning, head outside *without* your sunglasses and soak up the morning light for at least ten minutes. Aim for 5-10 minutes on a sunny day, and up to 20 minutes if it's overcast. Viewing sunlight within the first hours of waking increases early-day cortisol release, which promotes wakefulness and strengthens your immune system.[137] This morning light exposure also helps suppress lingering melatonin levels, enhancing alertness and preparing the body to fall asleep approximately 16 hours later.

Exposure to morning sunlight plays a crucial role in regulating our body's internal clock, known as the circadian rhythm. This is a powerful way to improve sleep quality, mood, and overall health. For an added benefit, take a morning walk in the sunlight without your sunglasses.

2. PRIORITIZE EVENING SUNLIGHT EXPOSURE.

Get outside at regular intervals throughout the day. Aim for at least an hour. Later in the day, the sun is lower in the sky, producing yellow and orange wavelengths that inform your body that it's time to begin relaxing and moving into the sleep phase. Even if you miss your morning sunlight viewing window, this second opportunity can still be useful in readjusting your circadian clock and reducing some of the negative effects of artificial light exposure at night.[138]

3. CONSIDER WEARING BLUE LIGHT-BLOCKING GLASSES.

A 2015 study investigated the effects of blue light–blocking glasses on adolescents exposed to light-emitting diode (LED) screens in the evening.[139] The findings revealed that participants who wore these glasses experienced reduced suppression of melatonin—a hormone that regulates sleep—compared to those who wore clear lenses. Additionally, the use of blue light–blocking glasses led to decreased alertness and increased sleepiness before bedtime. These results suggest that such glasses can mitigate the alerting effects of evening screen exposure, potentially improving sleep.

4. OPTIMIZE YOUR HEALTH WITH RED AND INFRARED LIGHT EXPOSURE.

These types of lights can penetrate tissues and enhance mitochondrial function, leading to improved skin health, wound healing, and potential neuroprotection. Additionally, red light exposure in the morning may support eye health and offset aging-related vision decline.[140] In the evening, using red light can promote alertness without disrupting sleep patterns.[141]

ENVIRONMENT

I. BRING NATURE INTO YOUR HOME OR OFFICE.

We can derive a lot of joy and benefit from the beauty that we take in. Surround yourself with a visually pleasing environment whenever possible. This can reduce stress levels, promote relaxation, and improve mood.[142] Bringing natural elements like sunlight and plants into our spaces can lower cortisol levels, the body's primary stress hormone, promoting relaxation and building resilience. You can start to enhance your visual environment one room at a time; begin by removing clutter and adding in color, natural light, and nature where you can.

2. STEP OUT INTO NATURE.

By spending just 20 minutes in nature, you can significantly decrease cortisol levels, which will impact your mental and physical health tremendously.[143] Natural elements, harmonious colors, and balanced designs engage our brain's visual processing centers, fostering a sense of calm and stability.

3. REDECORATE YOUR SPACE.

Intentionally designed aesthetic environments stimulate the release of dopamine, a neurotransmitter associated with pleasure and motivation. Incorporating vibrant colors and meaningful objects into our surroundings can boost mood, well-being, and creativity. This concept, known as "dopamine decor," emphasizes the intentional design of spaces to boost mood and cognitive function.[144]

By painting even one accent wall in the room, you can change the way your room feels. Bring in one beautiful object to accent your room - my go-to object is a beautifully potted plant - to gaze at and uplift your mood. Incorporating colors can also boost your creativity and productivity. While cluttered spaces can overstimulate the brain, leading to distraction and cognitive fatigue, attractive and organized environments encourage sustained focus and innovative thinking.

4. DRESS FOR LESS STRESS.

What we wear can also uplift our moods. How do you want to feel at any given moment? If you're going for professional and productive, be sure to wear something that helps you feel this way! Sporty and athletic? The same thing—put on a workout outfit that activates those feelings. Ready to create a cozy and relaxed environment? Choose soft fabrics and subdued colors to activate your relaxation response.

What colors put you in a good mood? Since discovering the dopamine-inducing power of colored clothing, I've had a lot of fun wearing bright jewel colors, even painting my nails and bringing in accessories to match. Gorgeous colors can brighten your visuals and brighten your mood! Be mindful of how comfortable fabrics and colors stimulate positive feelings and create a harmonious environment.

SCREEN TIME REDUCTION

I. MIND THE SCROLL HOLES.

Computer and device screens have become one of the biggest threats to mental well-being. Turn your screens on night mode where possible, and be mindful of your scrolling time, especially after dark.

2. SET A FOCUS TIMER TO LIMIT EXPOSURE.

To get the most out of your time online, set a focus timer. Turn off other distractions and focus solely on your work for 50 minutes. When your timer goes off, turn off your screen and move your body, hydrate, and step away for a break. By focusing on one task at a time and not allowing yourself to wander off into whatever pings, dings, and reminders you're being sent, you will take back control of your technology and put yourself into the driver's seat of your experience.

TOUCH

I. GROUND YOURSELF THROUGH TOUCH.

Grounding, or earthing, is the simple act of connecting your bare feet directly to the earth. Grounding can improve sleep, normalize cortisol rhythms, reduce pain, and shift the autonomic nervous system from sympathetic to parasympathetic activation.[145] To try it, sit, stand, or walk barefoot on grass, sand, or soil for 20–30 minutes, letting nature work its restorative magic.

2. USE YOUR HANDS.

I'll always remember the advice of my dear cousin Barb during a particularly prolonged period of depression after my first hospital stint in 2012. Barb is often busy with creative projects around the house and garden - baking sourdough bread, planting, harvesting, sewing, and cooking nutritious foods. Barb's advice to me was to start using my hands, specifically beginning with cleaning out a drawer.

Her advice helped me to realize that I had outsourced most of the handiwork in my life, and in doing so, I was depriving myself of potential brain-based satisfaction. Growing up in a culture that emphasized external achievement and professional success, I'm grateful to have reconnected with the deep power and purpose found in the simple, meaningful rhythms of home and garden. These often-overlooked acts of creation and care can offer profound satisfaction, grounding, and a renewed sense of thriving, reminding us that fulfillment isn't only found out there and in the sacred work of tending to what's right in front of us.

3. KEEP YOURSELF BUSY WITH CHORES OR CRAFTS.

While outsourcing house and garden work can be practical and timesaving, there can be tremendous therapeutic value in doing things with our hands. Using your hands engages the brain in physical, purposeful tasks, which can reduce stress and promote mindfulness. Activities like washing dishes or gardening stimulate sensory input and create a calming rhythm, fostering a meditative state.

Engage in a few minutes of using your hands throughout your week to see how it will make you feel. Engaging our mind and body through the hands can release tension, boost our mood, and provide the satisfaction of accomplishment.

4. MAKE USE OF MEAL PREPPING.

When we are open to it, using our hands to be creative and productive can bring a sense of accomplishment and enjoyment. Chopping produce or preparing a delicious meal can also trigger these feel-good chemical reactions inside our brains and bodies.

Set the scene for enjoyment - brew a cup of aromatic tea, simmer some onions and garlic on the stove, set the lights at a pleasant level, and turn on your favorite tunes to enhance the experience. **While the importance of homemaking has been downplayed in certain societies, when you consider the *profound* impact of food on our mental and overall health, *this sacred act can be restored to its true glory.***

SOUND

1. GET CURIOUS ABOUT SOUND HEALING.

Sound has incredible healing properties. You can use specific sound frequencies, rhythms, and music to alter your moods and boost emotional well-being. Ancient cultures have implemented sound healing practices for millennia, chanting, drumming, and playing tunes through sound bowls or animal horns, to name a few examples. You can utilize the power of sound to activate the parasympathetic nervous system to induce calmer feelings. Using a sound healing app can also provide your brain with a respite to recharge, focus, or relax.

2. SET THE MOOD WITH SOUND.

You can harness the power of sound to create your desired mood. Turning on a workout playlist can help you get motivated before and during a workout. Experiment with the songs and sounds that resonate with what you need, and as with all the upgrades we've discussed, stay present and mindful of what the music is bringing up for you and adjust your experience accordingly.

3. EXPLORE NEW TUNES OR RECONNECT WITH THE OLD.

When it comes to music, certain songs and melodies from our past are intrinsically connected in the mind with specific memories and associations from the past. Most people have a lasting preference for songs they enjoyed as adolescents and early adults. There's a phenomenon called the 'reminiscence bump,' which suggests that these songs evoke strong personal memories and emotional responses, which makes them enduring favorites. Be aware of what memories your music is bringing up for you.

Are these memories that you want to relive? If so, great - keep listening. If not, it's the perfect moment to explore new music and try to create new memories and associations for those songs. Whenever I go on a vacation or day trip with my husband, we listen to a new album or two over the course of the trip. This way, we create positive associations for the songs, and we get to relive our memories of the trip long after the trip ends.

SMELL

I. AROMATHERAPY

The sense of smell is a powerful yet overlooked tool to enhance our moods. Smell is closely linked to mood because it's directly linked to the brain's limbic system, which controls emotions and memory. Certain scents, like lavender and chamomile, can trigger the release of calming neurotransmitters like serotonin, reducing stress and promoting relaxation. Other scents, such as citrus and peppermint aromas, are known to stimulate the brain and boost energy or focus.

To enhance your mood, you can smell essential oils in a diffuser, light scented candles (opt for all-natural, non-toxic), sauté aromatic vegetables, or use a roll-on essential oil to tap into the power of scent on the go. Choose specific scents based on your goals, like lavender for relaxation, eucalyptus for invigoration, or vanilla for comfort, and allow your sense of smell to elevate your emotional state naturally.

2. ENJOY THE SWEET SMELL OF CLEAN AIR.

You can also bring herbs and other air-cleansing plants into your home environment. Herbs can be smelled and used in recipes and teas. As long as the plants are maintained, they will create a purer environment that will naturally smell cleaner.

TASTE

I. GET CURIOUS ABOUT FOOD.

Foods and the entire experience around eating have powerful associations with your life experiences. Childhood memories of eating certain foods on special occasions can make near-indelible marks. Each time we revisit a food or taste, we are also revisiting a memory. This is fine and good if these foods support your well-being. But if an upgrade in your nutrition is in order, give yourself time to go through the ECHO process, learning about, becoming curious about, and experimenting with the foods that will support your upgraded state of being. With the right amount of motivation to feel good and curiosity about your experience, you can learn to love all sorts of foods, even ones you've never tried.

2. EXPAND YOUR PALETTE.

When it comes to food, we cannot confuse short-term pleasure and enjoyment with long-term benefit. You *can* grow to enjoy nutritious foods as you're eating them, and yes, they will benefit you in the long run. But be careful when it comes to highly palatable, processed, overly sweet, or overly salty foods, as well as chemicals disguising themselves as food. As we've discussed, these food substitutes wreak havoc on the mind and body.

3. PRACTICE MINDFUL EATING.

The body's ability to adapt and learn to enjoy new food experiences is incredible. While it may feel like a loss for some people to decrease added sugars and other unfit foods, over time, the body becomes more highly attuned to the natural sweetness and rich bouquet of flavors in veggies, fruits, spices, and other nutrient-dense choices. Slowing down to sense the intricacies of a particular food through taste, texture, and scent can bring more pleasure to this experience.

4. FOCUS ON FOOD AS MEDICINE.

When you are giving your body the hydration, nutrients, and vitamins it needs, it's less likely to crave items that don't serve your health and wellness goals. Over time, you will recalibrate your taste buds and rebalance your body's sweetness and flavor perception.

INTUITION

I. HONOR YOUR OWN IDEAS AND FEELINGS.

Part of the healing process is getting in touch, or getting *back* in touch with your sixth sense: intuition. Over the course of our socialization, we can receive messages that are contrary to our intuition. It's easy for children to ignore or override their intuition and accept the advice of an adult, just as adult professionals override their intuition and common sense to obey authority. Similarly, it's logical that in the health journey, people can ignore their own intuition in favor of accepting professional advice.

I'm definitely not advocating for ignoring the right professional advice or the thoughtful input of other people on your journey. But I *am* advocating that you keep your Critical Insight in place, question the advice and motivations of other people, and make sure they're in line with your goals and best interests. Listening to your intuition means doing what you want on the deepest level and doing what's truly best for you.

If it is truly the best thing for you, ultimately, it is also going to be the best thing for the universe and all beings. To reconnect with your intuition, begin by taking a few slow breaths before making a decision. Quiet your mind, focus on your breath, and ask yourself, "What is going to be the best path forward at this moment?" Practice leaning into this intuition and make a note of what transpires when you do.

2. SLOW DOWN TO SENSE MORE.

One way to get in touch with your intuition, how you feel and what you want on the deepest levels, is to simply *slow down*. Step away from the input; put your phone down, take a break from other people, and give yourself fifteen minutes of quiet. Take some deep breaths and notice the thoughts in your mind without judging or critiquing yourself.

Notice whatever fears and motivations are swirling through your thoughts. As you breathe deeply, notice sensations in your body, taking special notice of the feelings in your midsection. Is your body reacting with tightness or openness? Are there unresolved questions that you need to answer before deciding? Once you have all the information at your fingertips, listen to how your body is reacting and how it is signaling you to respond.

3. KEEP IT SIMPLE.

Simple chores, like folding laundry, food prep, or washing dishes, require just enough attention to keep you focused and allow your mind to relax. This balance enables mental "wandering" that can help process emotions, solve problems, and spark creative ideas. If you've ever wondered why your best ideas come to you in the shower, this is the reason.

For people processing difficult memories or emotions, mental wandering can present challenges. Be mindful of what you need, and if it's a distraction for your own comfort, do what serves you best.

Consider how, with the right mindset, a simple chore can provide your mind with a much-needed reset and even spark joy! Building this into your day can improve your problem-solving potential, enhance your emotional regulation, and even boost creativity by allowing the brain to freely explore thoughts and connections in the background.

Keep in mind that slowing down can be difficult if you've got a negative thought track in the background, so be sure to revisit the ideas around mindfulness, non-judgmental awareness, and self-compassion can help you shift your thought tracks.

I hope you've enjoyed learning about the sensory healing protocols. You're all set and ready to begin testing these upgrades in your healing journey, and you've got the ECHO method in your pocket to use as you progress. By harnessing the power of our six senses, we can improve our mood, boost our energy, and create a more positive and fulfilling life.

CHAPTER 14 SUMMARY

KEY CONCEPTS

1. What you take in through the senses can impact your well-being. It can influence how you feel, think, and show up.

2. Your body is deeply connected to the natural world. From bringing in more natural light to adding a few grounding elements from nature into your space, these things make a difference. Nature can help regulate our rhythms and restore calm in our lives.

QUESTIONS

1. Take inventory of your surroundings and habits: the lighting, your screen habits, your wardrobe, even the space you live in. Is there anything that you feel inspired to shift or change in the coming days?

2. Consider your daily habits and routines for a moment. What could be some welcome additions to your day over the long term that could bring about a greater sense of well-being?

3. What colors, textures, materials, sounds, or scents help you feel more at ease and grounded? What's the most convenient way for you to bring more of them into your daily life?

FROM SILENCE AND SHAME TO SOLIDARITY AND STRENGTH

If I can do it, you can do it.

—Marsha Linehan, Creator of DBT

This book began with a tragic story—the moment I learned of 18-year-old Gila Hammer's death by suicide. The grief and shock were immense, but alongside that came a piercing realization: I could no longer stay silent about my story.

In the time since, I've come to understand just how many people are carrying similar pain. **Gila's struggle reflects a heartbreaking reality that's become far too common, especially among today's youth. In In 2023, the first leading cause of death among Americans under the age of 44 is "unintentional injury deaths," and the second leading cause of death is…. suicide.**[146] Accounting for death by overdose, in the first category, and for iatrogenic harm related accident prone behavior, the losses being incurred from mental health related causes tops anything else. This should be a wake-up call for all of us. And yet, silence still surrounds these conversations.

Healing doesn't come from silence. We've learned this the hard way. **Healing will come from the truth.** From courageous storytelling. From dissolving the shame that keeps people suffering in isolation. I've been cautioned several times by well-meaning people not to share my story so publicly. They've warned that it could damage my reputation. But here's what I know: If telling the truth helps even one person feel less alone, or if sharing my story gives someone the tools to take their next step forward, then it's worth it. Every. Single. Time. I made the conscious choice to speak up. And I hope you will ultimately do the same. Some people may not yet understand how urgent this work is. But I do. So I'll keep showing up—story in hand, voice steady, head held high. Here is the bottom line for me: human life is more important than opinions based in ignorance.

I can't rewrite the past, or erase the devastating statistics. But I can use my voice to declare—this mental health epidemic is not normal. We cannot stay silent, and we cannot normalize the staggering numbers that reflect our collective pain. We must normalize talking about today's mental health landscape, the information at our fingertips, and the ways in which we are able to move forward.

What liberated me—and gave me permission to finally share my story—was truth. When I realized I wasn't fundamentally flawed or disordered, as I had once been led to believe, everything shifted.

My hope is that the up and coming generations will carry the torch of truth—illuminating the roots of a mental health crisis that's burning like wild fire. We need ambassadors for a new tomorrow—voices brave enough to break the silence, hands steady enough to heal what's been harmed, and hearts bold enough to spark a renaissance of vitality among the overlooked and abandoned.

My blessing for you, is this: May truth be your compass and compassion your legacy. The future is unwritten—it belongs to those brave enough to speak the truth, imagine boldly, and build what's never been before. As Eleanor Roosevelt once said, *"The future belongs to those who believe in the beauty of their dreams."*

A healthy world is going to be the most beautiful thing we can imagine. Just think of a world where children grow up feeling whole expressing themselves honestly and authentically, and where seeking support is met with open arms, empowerment, and hope in humanity. A world where emotions are honored, not pathologized; where resilience is built through connection, not and not forced "correction." In this world, students will learn nervous system regulation, self care, and interpersonal relationship skills alongside math and reading. Communities will rally to support their members—not just in crisis, but in every day living. People will recognize that they are not defined or limited by the labels or beliefs applied to them by others, no matter how many credentials those people have collected.

This is the future we can dream of, and it is also the future that we can build. It begins now, with us. I believe that with God's help, we can reclaim the lives we've been granted and the wholeness we're here to embody. **We can protest a broken system—not just by holding up signs, but with our daily lives. By reclaiming our bodies, our minds, and our birthright to thrive—beyond diagnoses, beyond stigma, beyond limits that were never ours to begin with.**

As you've seen in these pages, healing isn't always linear. Sometimes it's messy. Sometimes it's slow. But it is always possible. With the right tools, aligned support, and a willingness to reconnect with your inner compass, the journey can be joyful, energizing, and transformational. This is your journey—and yes, it *is* possible.

In the words of Marsha Linehan—once severely disabled by mental illness and hospitalization in her youth, now a respected professor emeritus of psychology and the creator of Dialectical Behavior Therapy (DBT): **"If I can do it, you can do it."**

The path to wellness is lifelong. But it can be walked with purpose, and with hope, and we can feel progress from the outset. By tending to the core areas of your mental health—**Physiology, Psychology, People, and Purpose**—you can build a life that honors your whole self. This is how we will thrive.

I hope this book has brought you comfort, clarity, and the confidence to reimagine what's possible. May you feel empowered to make conscious, consistent upgrades to your mindset, your routines, your relationships, and your purpose. You deserve to feel well. You deserve to thrive.

If my journey or the information you've read here has served you in any way, I invite you to pass along this book to someone who could benefit from it. Share it. Talk about it. Recommend it to someone in need.

Be a spark. One story, one conversation, one act of courage can start a ripple effect that reaches far beyond what we can see.

Mental health science is still evolving—and so is my work. If you'd like to stay connected, explore the latest wellness research, or access additional resources, you can visit <u>www.mentalhealthreclaimed.com</u> and www.azijankovic.com.

My hope is to reach and support as many people as possible through the lessons and insights shared in this book. By engaging with these ideas—and by sharing your own—you can be part of the *Mental Health, Reclaimed* movement.

I believe that when we dare to embrace every part of ourselves—flawed, beautiful, in-process—we unlock the strength and peace that come from taking radical responsibility for our lives.

This is your journey now.

Personal.

Powerful.

And full of possibility.

Let's rise, and let's thrive.

Onwards—together.

ENDNOTES

1. Calati, R., Ferrari, C., Brittner, M., Oasi, O., Olié, E., Carvalho, A. F., & Courtet, P. (2019). Social isolation and suicide risk: A literature review and perspectives. *European Psychiatry, 56,* 78-92.

2. Solmi, M., Radua, J., Olivola, M., Croce, E., Soardo, L., Salazar de Pablo, G., ... & Fusar-Poli, P. (2023). Age of onset and cumulative risk of mental disorders: A cross-national analysis of population surveys from 29 countries. *The Lancet Psychiatry, 10*(10), 790–800.

3. GBD 2019 Mental Disorders Collaborators. (2022). Global, regional, and national burden of 12 mental disorders in 204 countries and territories, 1990–2019: A systematic analysis for the Global Burden of Disease Study 2019. *The Lancet Psychiatry, 9*(2), 137–150.

4. Omondi, K. (2024). Mental health stigma and its impact on help-seeking behavior. *International Journal of Humanity and Social Sciences, 3*(3), 15–29.

5. Adams, K. M., Butsch, W. S., & Kohlmeier, M. (2015). The state of nutrition education at US medical schools. *Journal of Biomedical Education,* 2015, Article ID 357627

6. Singh, B., Olds, T., Curtis, R., Dumuid, D., Virgara, R., Watson, A., ... & Kandola, A. (2023). *Effectiveness of physical activity interventions for improving depression, anxiety and distress: An overview of systematic reviews. British Journal of Sports Medicine, 57*(12), 865–875

7. Porges, S. W. (2011). *The polyvagal theory: Neurophysiological foundations of emotions, attachment, communication, and self-regulation. Frontiers in Human Neuroscience, 5,* 1–15.

8. Kok, B. E., & Fredrickson, B. L. (2013). *Upward spirals of the heart: Autonomic flexibility, as indexed by vagal tone, reciprocally and prospectively predicts positive emotions and social connectedness. Psychological Science, 24*(7), 1123–1132.

9. Benedetti, F., & Amanzio, M. (2011). The placebo response: How words and rituals change the patient's brain. *Neuroscience, 6*(1), 1–10.

10. Radiology error statistics: Berlin, L. (2007). Accuracy of diagnostic procedures: Has it improved over the past five decades? *American Journal of Roentgenology, 188(5),* 1173–1178

11. Harvey, A. G. (2008). Sleep and circadian rhythms in bipolar disorder: Seeking synchrony, harmony, and regulation. *American Journal of Psychiatry,* 165(7), 820–829.

12. Lewy, A. J., Lefler, B. J., Emens, J. S., & Bauer, V. K. (2006). The circadian basis of winter depression. *Proceedings of the National Academy of Sciences,* 103(19), 7414–7419.

13. Moncrieff, J. (2014). The bipolar epidemic. *Joanna Moncrieff.*

14. Airainer, M., & Seifert, R. (2024). Lithium, the gold standard drug for bipolar disorder: Analysis of current clinical studies. *Naunyn-Schmiedeberg's Archives of Pharmacology, 397,* 9723–9743.

15. Moncrieff, J. (2015, July 1). Reasons not to believe in lithium. *Joanna Moncrieff's Blog.* https://joannamoncrieff.com/2015/07/01/reasons-not-to-believe-in-lithium/

16. Prescription stats: Centers for Disease Control and Prevention. (2023). QuickStats: Percentage of adults aged ≥18 years who took prescription medication during the past 12 months, by sex and age group — National Health Interview Survey, United States, 2021. *Morbidity and Mortality Weekly Report,* 72(16), 450.

17. Four or more prescriptions: Kaiser Family Foundation. (2023). Public opinion on prescription drugs and their prices. Retrieved from https://www.kff.org/other/poll-finding/public-opinion-on-prescription-drugs-and-their-prices/

18. Storey, D. (2024, April 30). *Mental health diagnoses take unprecedented leap.* Psychiatrist.com. https://www.psychiatrist.com/news/mental-health-diagnoses-take-unprecedented-leap/

19. Centers for Disease Control and Prevention. (2024, April 22). *Fast facts: Health and economic costs of chronic conditions.* U.S. Department of Health & Human Services. https://www.cdc.gov/chronic-disease/data-research/facts-stats/index.html

20. Centers for Disease Control and Prevention. (2024, June 3). *Mental health: Chronic disease indicators.* U.S. Department of Health & Human Services. https://www.cdc.gov/cdi/indicator-definitions/mental-health.html

21. HMO and diminishing quality healthcare: American Family Physician. (2011). House Calls. *American Family Physician,* 83(8), 925. Retrieved from https://www.aafp.org/pubs/afp/issues/2011/0415/p925.html

22. PBMs: Federal Trade Commission. (2024). *Pharmacy Benefit Managers: The Powerful Middlemen Inflating Drug Costs and Squeezing Main Street Pharmacies.* Retrieved from https://www.ftc.gov/reports/pharmacy-benefit-managers-report

23. Purdue Scandal: AMA Journal of Ethics. (2020). How FDA Failures Contributed to the Opioid Crisis. *AMA Journal of Ethics,* 22(8), E743-750. Retrieved from https://journalofethics.ama-assn.org/article/how-fda-failures-contributed-opioid-crisis/2020-08

24. Berg, P. (Director). (2023). *Painkiller* [Television series]. Netflix.

25. Medical Bankruptcy: The American Journal of Medicine. (2009). Medical Bankruptcy in the United States, 2007: Results of a National Study. *The American Journal of Medicine, 122*(8), 741-746. Retrieved from https://www. amjmed.com/article/S0002-9343(09)00525-7/fulltext

26. Medical Entrepreneur turned advocate: Rogan, J. (Host). (2024, October 1). #2208 – *Brigham Buhler* [Audio podcast episode]. In *The Joe Rogan Experience*. Spotify. https://open.spotify.com/episode/42LICozR75ovDHVHLxazy1

27. Cosgrove, L., & Krimsky, S. (2012). A comparison of DSM-IV and DSM-5 panel members' financial associations with industry: A pernicious problem persists. *PLoS Medicine, 9*(3), e1001190.

28. DSM and APA funding: BioSpace. (2022, November 16). *DSM-5 panel members received $14.2M in industry funding: Study.* Retrieved from https://www. biospace.com/dsm-5-panel-members-received-14-2m-in-industry-funding-study

29. Mad in America. (2017, January 10). *Allen Frances and the "Overdiagnosing" of Children.* Retrieved from https://www.madinamerica.com/2017/01/ allen-frances-overdiagnosing-children/

30. Diagnostic inflation: Mad in America. (2017, January 10). *Allen Frances and the "Overdiagnosing" of Children.* Retrieved from https://www.madinamerica. com/2017/01/allen-frances-overdiagnosing-children/

31. Mad in America. (2017, January 10). *Allen Frances and the "Overdiagnosing" of Children.* Retrieved from https://www.madinamerica.com/2017/01/ allen-frances-overdiagnosing-children/

32. Hughes, P. M., Annis, I. E., McGrath, R. E., & Thomas, K. C. (2024). Psychotropic medication prescribing across medical providers, 2016–2019. *Psychiatric Services, 75*(5), 477–480.

33. Hofling, C. K., Brotzman, E., Dalrymple, S., Graves, N., & Pierce, C. M. (1966). *An experimental study of nurse-physician relationships. Journal of Nervous and Mental Disease, 143*(2), 171–180

34. Birney, M. E., Reicher, S. D., & Haslam, S. A. (2024). Obedience as "Engaged Followership": A review and research agenda. *Philosophia Scientiæ, 28*(2), 91–105.

35. Dweck, C. S. (2006). *Mindset: The new psychology of success.* Random House.

36. Eger, E. E. (2019, June 24). *Super Soul Special: Dr. Edith Eva Eger: The Choice* [Audio podcast episode]. In O. Winfrey (Host), *Super Soul.* Oprah.com

37. Eger, E. E. (2017). *The choice: Embrace the possible.* Simon & Schuster.

38. Neff, K. (2011). *Self-compassion: The proven power of being kind to yourself.* HarperCollins.

39. Ferrari, M., Hunt, C., Harrysunker, A., Abbott, M. J., Beath, A. P., & Einstein, D. A. (2019). Self-compassion interventions and psychosocial outcomes: A meta-analysis of RCTs. *Mindfulness, 10*(8), 1455–1473.

40. Kim, S., Thibodeau, R., & Jorgensen, R. S. (2011). Shame, guilt, and depressive symptoms: A meta-analytic review. *Psychological Bulletin, 137*(1), 68–96

41. Mayo Clinic. (2019). Cognitive behavioral therapy. In *Tests and Procedures.*

42. Mindfulness: Hölzel, B. K., Carmody, J., Vangel, M., Congleton, C., Yerramsetti, S. M., Gard, T., & Lazar, S. W. (2011). Mindfulness practice leads to increases in regional brain gray matter density. *Psychiatry Research: Neuroimaging, 191*(1), 36–43.

43. Tang, Y. Y., et al. (2015). The neuroscience of mindfulness meditation.

44. Kaliman, P., Álvarez-López, M. J., Cosín-Tomás, M., Rosenkranz, M. A., Lutz, A., & Davidson, R. J. (2014). Rapid changes in histone deacetylases and inflammatory gene expression in expert meditators. *Psychoneuroendocrinology, 40*, 96–107.

45. Porges, S. W. (2011). *The polyvagal theory: Neurophysiological foundations of emotions, attachment, communication, and self-regulation.* New York: W.W. Norton & Company.

46. Bandura, A. (1997). *Self-Efficacy: The Exercise of Control.*

47. Brain Energy Budget: Raichle, M. E., & Gusnard, D. A. (2002). Appraising the brain's energy budget. *Proceedings of the National Academy of Sciences, 99*(16), 10237–10239.

48. Robbins, A. (1991). *Awaken the giant within: How to take immediate control of your mental, emotional, physical and financial destiny!* Free Press.

49. Agouti Mice: Dolinoy, D. C. (2008). The agouti mouse model: An epigenetic biosensor for nutritional and environmental alterations on the fetal epigenome. *Nutrition Reviews, 66*(Suppl 1), S7–S11.

50. Klibaner-Schiff, E., Simonin, E. M., Akdis, C. A., Cheong, A., Johnson, M. M., Karagas, M. R., Kirsh, S., Kline, O., Mazumdar, M., Oken, E., Sampath, V., Vogler, N., Wang, X., & Nadeau, K. C. (2024). Environmental exposures influence multigenerational epigenetic transmission. *Clinical Epigenetics, 16*(1), 145.

51. Fitzgerald, K. N., Hodges, R., Hanes, D., Stack, E., Cheishvili, D., Szyf, M., ... & Bhasin, M. K. (2023). Potential reversal of epigenetic age using a diet and lifestyle intervention: a pilot randomized clinical trial. *Aging, 15*

52. Nad.com. (2023, October). *Harvard study reveals that omega-3s, vitamin D, and exercise additively slow biological aging.*

53. Zubieta, J.-K., Bueller, J. A., Jackson, L. R., Scott, D. J., Xu, Y., Koeppe, R. A., & Stohler, C. S. (2005). Placebo effects mediated by endogenous opioid activity on μ-opioid receptors. *Journal of Neuroscience, 25*(34), 7754–7762.

54. Prabakar, A. D. (2024). The power of thought: The role of psychological attentiveness and emotional support in patient trajectories. *The Yale Journal of Biology and Medicine, 97*(3), 335–347.

55. Flegal, K. M., Carroll, M. D., Ogden, C. L., & Johnson, C. L. (2002). Prevalence and trends in obesity among US adults, 1999-2000. *JAMA, 288*(14), 1723–1727.

56. Sánchez-Villegas, A., Verberne, L., De Irala, J., Ruíz-Canela, M., Toledo, E., Serra-Majem, L., & Martínez-González, M. A. (2011). Dietary fat intake and the risk of depression: The SUN Project. PLoS One, 6(1), e16268.

57. Zhang, L., Sun, H., Liu, Z., Yang, J., & Liu, Y. (2024). Association between dietary sugar intake and depression in US adults: a cross-sectional study using data from the National Health and Nutrition Examination Survey 2011–2018. BMC Psychiatry, 24, Article 110.

58. Cigarette Plain Packaging: PR Newswire. (2024, January 17). *Tobacco plain packaging progress continues worldwide, with 42 countries and territories moving forward with regulations.* PR Newswire.

59. R.J. Reynolds Tobacco Company. (1946). *More doctors smoke Camels than any other cigarette* [Advertisement]. *Ladies' Home Journal.*

60. Kearns, C. E., Schmidt, L. A., & Glantz, S. A. (2016). Sugar industry and coronary heart disease research: A historical analysis of internal industry documents. *JAMA Internal Medicine, 176*(11), 1680–1685.

61. Nguyen, K. H., Glantz, S. A., Palmer, C. N., & Schmidt, L. A. (2020). Transferring racial/ethnic marketing strategies from tobacco to food corporations: Philip Morris and Kraft General Foods. American Journal of Public Health, 110(3), 329–336.

62. Huberman, A. D. (Host). (2021, April 19). *How our hormones control our hunger, eating & satiety* [Audio podcast episode]. In *Huberman Lab.*

63. Taubes, G. (2016). *The case against sugar.* New York: Alfred A. Knopf.

64. Zhang, L., Sun, H., Liu, Z., Yang, J., & Liu, Y. (2024). Association between dietary sugar intake and depression in US adults: a cross-sectional study using data from the National Health and Nutrition Examination Survey 2011–2018. *BMC Psychiatry, 24*, Article 110.

65. Sugar crashes and anxiety, blood glucose instability: Means, C. (2024). *Stable blood sugar strategies, an easy grain-free tortilla recipe, and dry January recap.* Casey Means. https://www.caseymeans.com/learn/articles-newsletter-stable-blood-sugar-strategies-an-easy-grain-free-tortilla-recipe-and-dry-january-recap

66. Means, C. (2024). *Stable blood sugar strategies, an easy grain-free tortilla recipe, and dry January recap.* Casey Means. Retrieved May 8, 2025, from https://www.caseymeans.com/learn/articles-newsletter-stable-blood-sugar-strategies-an-easy-grain-free-tortilla-recipe-and-dry-january-recap

67. *Hidden in plain sight.* University of California, San Francisco. Retrieved from https://sugarscience.ucsf.edu/hidden-in-plain-sight/

68. *Hidden in plain sight.* University of California, San Francisco. Retrieved from https://sugarscience.ucsf.edu/hidden-in-plain-sight/

69. World Health Organization. (2015). *Guideline: Sugars intake for adults and children.* World Health Organization. Retrieved from https://www.who.int/publications/i/item/9789241549028

70. Lustig, R. H., Mulligan, K., Noworolski, S. M., Tai, V. W., Wen, M. J., Erkin-Cakmak, A., ... & Schwarz, J. M. (2016). Isocaloric fructose restriction and metabolic improvement in children with obesity and metabolic syndrome. *Obesity*, 24(2), 453-460.

71. Cogswell, M. E., Gunn, J. P., Yuan, K., Park, S., Merritt, R., & Galuska, D. A. (2021). Added sugars in school meals and the diets of school-age children. *Nutrients*, 13(2), 471.

72. World Health Organization. (n.d.). *Depression*. World Health Organization. Retrieved from https://www.who.int/news-room/fact-sheets/detail/depression

73. Centers for Disease Control and Prevention. (2023). National, state-level, and county-level prevalence of depression among adults — United States, 2020. *Morbidity and Mortality Weekly Report*, 72(24), 634–640.

74. World Population Review. (2024). *Sugar consumption by country 2024*. Retrieved from https://worldpopulationreview.com/country-rankings/sugar-consumption-by-country

75. Lustig, R. H. (n.d.). *Food addiction*. Robert Lustig. Retrieved from https://robertlustig.com/food-addiction/

76. Fuchs, M. (2022, January 25). *How to get healthier dopamine highs*. TIME. https://time.com/6155109/healthier-dopamine-highs/

77. Serotonin science: Nationwide Children's Hospital. (2023, February 28). *Dopamine and serotonin: Our own happy chemicals*. Nationwide Children's Hospital.

78. Yano, J. M., Yu, K., Donaldson, G. P., Shastri, G. G., Ann, P., Ma, L., Nagler, C. R., Ismagilov, R. F., Mazmanian, S. K., & Hsiao, E. Y. (2015). Indigenous bacteria from the gut microbiota regulate host serotonin biosynthesis. *Cell*, 161(2), 264–276.

79. Volkow, N. D., Wang, G. J., Fowler, J. S., & Telang, F. (2008). Overlapping neuronal circuits in addiction and obesity: Evidence of systems pathology. *Philosophical Transactions of the Royal Society B: Biological Sciences*, 363(1507), 3191–3200.

80. Gesch, C. B., Hammond, S. M., Hampson, S. E., Eves, A., & Crowder, M. J. (2002). Influence of supplementary vitamins, minerals and essential fatty acids on the antisocial behaviour of young adult prisoners: Randomised, placebo-controlled trial. *The British Journal of Psychiatry*, 181(1), 22–28.

81. Meridian Health Clinic. (n.d.). *How Rockefeller created the business of Western medicine*. https://meridianhealthclinic.com/how-rockefeller-created-the-business-of-western-medicine/

82. Diets don't work: The Ohio State University Wexner Medical Center. (n.d.). *That diet probably didn't work*. Health.osu.edu.

83. Centers for Disease Control and Prevention. (2001). *Duration of office visits to physicians: United States, 1997–98*. National Center for Health Statistics. Retrieved from https://stacks.cdc.gov/view/cdc/64035

84. Beck, A. T., Ward, C. H., Mendelson, M., Mock, J., & Erbaugh, J. (1961). An inventory for measuring depression. *Archives of General Psychiatry, 4*(6), 561–571.

85. Habets, M. F., van der Aa, L. M., & de Wit, N. J. W. (2022). Exploring the serotonin⊠probiotics⊠gut health axis: A review of evidence from studies with rodents and humans. *Food Science & Nutrition,* 10(4), 1000–1015.

86. Sarkar, A., Lehto, S. M., Harty, S., Moeller, A. H., Dinan, T. G., Cryan, J. F., & Burnet, P. W. J. (2016). Psychobiotics and the Manipulation of Bacteria–Gut–Brain Signals. *Trends in Neurosciences, 39*(11), 763–781

87. Sarkar, A., Lehto, S. M., Harty, S., Moeller, A. H., Dinan, T. G., Cryan, J. F., & Burnet, P. W. J. (2016). Psychobiotics and the Manipulation of Bacteria–Gut–Brain Signals. *Trends in Neurosciences, 39*(11), 763–781.

88. Carabotti, M., Scirocco, A., Maselli, M. A., & Severi, C. (2015). The gut-brain axis: Interactions between enteric microbiota, central and enteric nervous systems. *Annals of Gastroenterology, 28*(2), 203–209.

89. Moncrieff, J., Cooper, R. E., Stockmann, T., Amendola, S., Hengartner, M. P., & Horowitz, M. A. (2022). The serotonin theory of depression: A systematic umbrella review of the evidence. *Molecular Psychiatry, 27*(5), 2217–2229.

90. ibid

91. Moncrieff, J. (2023, June 21). *Contradictory responses to our review of serotonin and depression.* Retrieved from https://joannamoncrieff.com/2023/06/21/contradictory-responses-to-our-review-of-serotonin-and-depression/

92. Palmer, C. M. (2022). *Brain Energy: A Revolutionary Breakthrough in Understanding Mental Health—and Improving Treatment for Anxiety, Depression, OCD, PTSD, and More.* BenBella Books.

93. Cleveland Clinic. (n.d.). *Antipsychotic medications: Uses, common brands, and side effects.*

94. Cleveland Clinic. (2023, August 28). *Ketosis.* https://my.clevelandclinic.org/health/articles/24003-ketosis

95. Palmer, C. M. (2022). *Brain energy: A revolutionary breakthrough in understanding mental health—and improving treatment for anxiety, depression, OCD, PTSD, and more.* BenBella Books.

96. Maayan L, Correll CU. Management of antipsychotic-related weight gain. Expert Rev Neurother. 2010 Jul;10(7):1175-200.

97. Tidball, J. G. (2005). Inflammatory processes in muscle injury and repair. *American Journal of Physiology-Regulatory, Integrative and Comparative Physiology, 288*(2), R345–R353.

98. Furman, D., Campisi, J., Verdin, E., Carrera-Bastos, P., Targ, S., Franceschi, C., ... & Slavich, G. M. (2019). Chronic inflammation in the etiology of disease across the life span. *Nature Medicine, 25*(12), 1822–1832.

99. Bercik, P., Verdu, E. F., Foster, J. A., Macri, J., Potter, M., Huang, X., Malinowski, P., Jackson, W., Blennerhassett, P., Neufeld, K. A., Lu, J., Khan, W. I., Corthesy-Theulaz, I., Cherbut, C., Bergonzelli, G. E., & Collins, S. M. (2010). Chronic gastrointestinal inflammation induces anxiety-like behavior and alters central nervous system biochemistry in mice. *Gastroenterology, 139*(6), 2102–2112.e1.

100. Liu, X., Cao, S., & Zhang, X. (2022). Dietary inflammatory potential and the incidence of depression and anxiety: A meta-analysis of observational studies. *Frontiers in Nutrition, 9*, 930685.

101. Sherpa, N. N., De Giorgi, R., & Ostinelli, E. G. (2025). Efficacy and safety profile of oral creatine monohydrate in add-on to cognitive-behavioural therapy in depression: An 8-week pilot double-blind randomised placebo-controlled feasibility and exploratory trial in an under-resourced area. *European Neuropsychopharmacology, 93*, 15–16.

102. Fort Worth Wellness. (2024). *The dangers of seed oils: Insights from leading experts.* Fort Worth Wellness. https://www.fortworthwellness.net/post/the-dangers-of-seed-oils-insights-from-leading-experts

103. National Institutes of Health. (2014). Single episode of binge drinking linked to gut leakage and immune system effects. Retrieved from https://www.nih.gov/news-events/news-releases/single-episode-binge-drinking-linked-gut-leakage-immune-system-effects

104. Barbuti, M., Menculini, G., Verdolini, N., Pacchiarotti, I., Kotzalidis, G. D., Tortorella, A., Vieta, E., & Perugi, G. (2023). A systematic review of manic/hypomanic and depressive switches in patients with bipolar disorder in naturalistic settings: The role of antidepressant and antipsychotic drugs. *European Neuropsychopharmacology, 73*, 1–15.

105. Waters, F., Chiu, V., Atkinson, A., & Blom, J. D. (2018). Severe sleep deprivation causes hallucinations and a gradual progression toward psychosis with increasing time awake. *Frontiers in Psychiatry, 9*, 303.

106. Statista Research Department. (2023, November). *Ideal number of hours of sleep according to adults in the United States as of 2023.* Statista.

107. Put Down the Vacuum: The Atlantic. (2024, November). *Why Women Can't Put Down the Vacuum.* Retrieved from https://www.theatlantic.com/ideas/archive/2024/11/why-women-cant-put-down-the-vacuum/680714/

108. Phillips, A. J. K., Clerx, W. M., O'Brien, C. S., Sano, A., Barger, L. K., Picard, R. W., & Lockley, S. W. (2023). Sleep regularity is a stronger predictor of mortality risk than sleep duration. *Sleep, 46*(1), zsac285.

109. Night owls and diagnoses: Stanford Medicine News Center. (2024, May). *Night owl behavior could hurt mental health, sleep study finds.*

110. Yetish, G., Kaplan, H., Gurven, M., Wood, B., Pontzer, H., Manger, P. R., Wilson, C., McGregor, R., & Siegel, J. M. (2015). Natural sleep and its seasonal variations in three pre-industrial societies. *Current Biology, 25*(21), 2862–2868.

111. Schuch, F. B., Vancampfort, D., Firth, J., Rosenbaum, S., Ward, P. B., Reichert, T., Bagatini, T., & Stubbs, B. (2023). Exercise as medicine for depressive symptoms? A systematic review and meta-analysis with meta-regression. *British Journal of Sports Medicine, 57*(16), 1049–1056.

112. Yu, Q., Wong, K.-K., Lei, O.-K., Nie, J., Shi, Q., Zou, L., & Kong, Z. (2022). Comparative effectiveness of multiple exercise interventions in the treatment of mental health disorders: A systematic review and network meta-analysis. *Sports Medicine - Open, 8*(1), 114.

113. Haines MS, Dichtel LE, Santoso K, Torriani M, Miller KK, Bredella MA. Association between muscle mass and insulin sensitivity independent of detrimental adipose depots in young adults with overweight/obesity. Int J Obes (Lond). 2020 Sep;44(9):1851-1858.

114. Means, C. (2024). *Good energy: The surprising connection between metabolism and mental health.* Penguin Press.

115. Target heart rate calculation: Means, C., & Means, C. (2024). *Good energy: The surprising connection between metabolism and limitless health.* Penguin Random House.

116. Shaking and Dancing Therapy: Gordon, J. S. (n.d.). *Breathe, Shake, Dance.* The Center for Mind-Body Medicine

117. Willpower and the brain: Teach RARE. (2023). *The Anterior Mid-Cingulate Cortex.* Retrieved from https://teachrare.org/the-anterior-mid-cingulate-cortex/

118. Huberman, A. (n.d.). *Tools to manage dopamine and improve motivation and drive.* Huberman Lab. Retrieved from https://www.hubermanlab.com/newsletter/tools-to-manage-dopamine-and-improve-motivation-and-drive

119. Huberman, A. [@hubermanlab]. (2024, April 15). *Use intermittent rewards to stay motivated* [Video]. Instagram. https://www.instagram.com/reel/DIDCXpZpkWF/

120. TIME. (2024, September 9). Is friendship therapy the next big thing in mental health? Retrieved from https://time.com/7014493/what-is-friendship-therapy/

121. U.S. Department of Health and Human Services. (2023). *Our epidemic of loneliness and isolation: The U.S. Surgeon General's advisory on the healing effects of social connection and community.*

122. **Waldinger, R. J., & Schulz, M. S.** (2023). *The good life: Lessons from the world's longest scientific study of happiness.* Simon & Schuster.

123. **Giles, H. (Ed.).** (2016). *Communication accommodation theory: Negotiating personal relationships and social identities across contexts.* Cambridge University Press.

124. Kovács, B., & Kleinbaum, A. M. (2019). Language-style similarity and social networks. *Psychological Science, 30*(3), 365–377.

125. Voss, C. (n.d.). Chris Voss Teaches the Art of Negotiation. MasterClass. Retrieved from https://www.masterclass.com/classes/chris-voss-teaches-the-art-of-negotiation/chapters/mirroring

126. Acquire a friend: Pirkei Avot 1:6. (n.d.). In *Sefaria.* Retrieved February 3, 2025, from https://www.sefaria.org/Pirkei_Avot.1.6

127. Peel, R., & Caltabiano, N. (2021). The relationship sabotage scale: An evaluation of factor analyses and construct validity. *BMC Psychology, 9*(1), 1-12.

128. Slavich GM. Social Safety Theory: A Biologically Based Evolutionary Perspective on Life Stress, Health, and Behavior. Annu Rev Clin Psychol. 2020 May 7;16:265-295.

129. Harvard Health Publishing. (2022, March 1). Understanding the stress response. *Harvard Health Publishing.*

130. Harvard Health Publishing. (2010, December 1). The health benefits of strong relationships. *Harvard Health Publishing*

131. This story was originally published in my first book; Jankovic, A. (2019). *Beyond all things: Insights to awaken joy, purpose, and spiritual connection.*

132. Devorah Benarouch, still a good friend to this day, has always inspired me with her devotion to doing acts of kindness and service.

133. Kook, A. I. (n.d.). *Souls* (Orot HaKodesh I, pp. 83–84).

134. Berger, A. (2025, April 11). *I kept my freedom in Hamas's captivity. The Wall Street Journal.* https://www.wsj.com/opinion/i-kept-my-freedom-in-hamas-captivity-passover-hostage-israel-gaza-27e85953

135. Jankovic, A. (Host). (2020, April 2). EP 31: Rabbi Abraham Twerski, MD. - Words of Encouragement and Wisdom to Meet any of Life's Challenges . In *Mental Health, RECLAIMED. with Dr. Azi Jankovic and Friends* [Audio podcast episode]. Apple Podcasts.

136. Witt-Doerring, J. (n.d.). *What is akathisia? The worst side effect of any psychiatric medication.* Taper Clinic. Retrieved May 8, 2025, from https://taperclinic.com/what-is-akathisia-the-worst-side-effect-of-any-psychiatric-medication/

137. Huberman, A. (2025). Using light for health. *Huberman Lab.* https://www.hubermanlab.com/newsletter/using-light-for-healthDexa+3Huberman Lab+3Dexa+3

138. Czeisler, C. A., & Gooley, J. J. (2007). Sleep and circadian rhythms in humans. *Cold Spring Harbor Symposia on Quantitative Biology, 72,* 579–597.

139. van der Lely, S., Frey, S., Garbazza, C., Wirz-Justice, A., Jenni, O. G., Steiner, R., ... & Schmidt, C. (2015). Blue blocker glasses as a countermeasure for alerting effects of evening light-emitting diode screen exposure in male teenagers. *The Journal of Adolescent Health, 56*(1), 113–119.

140. Umino Y, Denda M. Effect of red light on epidermal proliferation and mitochondrial activity. Skin Res Technol. 2023 Sep;29(9):e13447. doi: 10.1111/srt.13447. PMID: 37753678; PMCID: PMC10462800.

141. Figueiro MG, Sahin L, Wood B, Plitnick B. Light at Night and Measures of Alertness and Performance: Implications for Shift Workers. Biol Res Nurs. 2016 Jan;18(1):90-100.

142. Dijkstra, K., Pieterse, M., & Pruyn, A. (2008). Stress-reducing effects of indoor plants in the built healthcare environment: The mediating role of perceived attractiveness. *Preventive Medicine, 47*(3), 279–283.

143. Hunter, M. R., Gillespie, B. W., & Chen, S. Y.-P. (2019). Urban nature experiences reduce stress in the context of daily life based on salivary biomarkers. *Frontiers in Psychology, 10,* 722.

144. Ishizu, T., & Zeki, S. (2011). Toward a brain-based theory of beauty. PLoS ONE, 6(7), e21852.

145. Chevalier, G., Sinatra, S. T., Oschman, J. L., Sokal, K., & Sokal, P. (2015). The effects of grounding (earthing) on inflammation, the immune response, wound healing, and prevention and treatment of chronic inflammatory and autoimmune diseases. *Journal of Inflammation Research, 8,* 83–96.

146. Centers for Disease Control and Prevention. (2023). *WISQARS™—Animated leading causes of death.* National Center for Injury Prevention and Control. https://wisqars.cdc.gov/animated-leading-causes/